The Wellness Rx

DR. TAUB'S
7 DAY PROGRAM
FOR RADIANT
HEALTH & ENERGY

Edward A. Taub, M.D.

PRENTICE HALL
Englewood Cliffs, New Jersey 07632

Prentice-Hall International (UK) Limited, *London*
Prentice-Hall of Australia Pty. Limited, *Sydney*
Prentice-Hall Canada, Inc., *Toronto*
Prentice-Hall Hispanoamericana, S.A., *Mexico*
Prentice-Hall of India Private Limited, *New Delhi*
Prentice-Hall of Japan, Inc., *Tokyo*
Simon & Schuster Asia Pte. Ltd., *Singapore*
Editora Prentice-Hall do Brasil, Ltda., *Rio de Janeiro*

© 1994 by
Edward A. Taub, M.D.

This book is a reference work based on research by the author. The opinions
expressed herein are not necessarily those of or endorsed by the publisher. The
directions stated in this book are in no way to be considered as a substitute for
consultation with a duly licensed doctor.

10 9 8 7 6 5 4 3 2 1

Library of Congress Cataloging-in-Publication Data

Taub, Edward A.
   The Wellness Rx : Dr. Taub's 7-day program for
radiant health and energy / Edward A. Taub.
      p.   cm.
   Includes index.
   ISBN 0-13-082471-2. – ISBN 0-13-082463-1 (pbk.)
   1. Holistic medicine.   2. Health.   I. Title.
R733.T38   1994
613–dc20   94-7752
                                               CIP

ISBN 0-13-082471-2

ISBN 0-13-082463-1 (PBK.)

 PRENTICE HALL
Career & Personal Development
Englewood Cliffs, NJ 07632

Simon & Schuster, A Paramount Communications Company

Printed in the United States of America

Acknowledgments

To the author-physicians whose shoulders I climbed: Herbert Benson, M.D., Paul Brenner, M.D., Deepak Chopra, M.D., Larry Dossey, M.D., Tom Ferguson, M.D., Stanley E. Greben, M.D., Gerald G. Jampolsky, M.D., W. Brugh Joy, M.D., Melvin Konner, M.D., Steven Locke, M.D., John McDougall, M.D., Emmett Miller, M.D., Irving Oyle, M.D., Dean Ornish, M.D., M. Scott Peck, M.D., Karl Pribram, M.D., Rachel Naomi Remen, M.D., Samuel H. Sandweiss, M.D., Jonas Salk, M.D., Norman Shealy, M.D., Bernie S. Siegel, M.D., O. Carl Simonton, M.D., Lendon Smith, M.D., John Travis, M.D.

To members of the National Advisory Board of the Wellness Medicine Institute: Harold Bloomfield, M.D., Joycelyn Elders, M.D., Stanley Greben, M.D., Robert Lubell, D.D.S., Ron Myers, Senator Paul Simon, John Smith, M.D., Ron Pion, M.D., Marc Ungar, Phil Gower.

To the wonderful citizens of Mt. Carmel, Illinois and to my Community Advisory Board: Bill Hackler, Bank President; Harry Benson, College President; Pastor Bob Killion, Methodist Minister; Father Clyde Grogan, Catholic Priest; John Nolan, Financial Advisor; Steve Schwartz, Educator; Hytham Beck, Physician and Surgeon.

To Edward V. Fritzky, Jeff Hoyak, Gary Lauger, Pat F. Iaschetti and the PROSTEP Team at Lederle Laboratories for helping to save Mt. Carmel's children.

To my original helpers: Sidney Adler, M.D., Martin Baren, M.D., Merlin DuVal, M.D., Joel Elkes, M.D., Charles Kleeman, M.D., Julius Richmond, M.D., Jacques Soudjian, M.D., Paul Wehrle, M.D.

To the creative genius of Tim Bahr, Meagan Walker and the dedicated team at Orbis Production for "The National Wellness Stop Smoking Campaign."

To my son Marc Taub, M.D., and my brother Lanny Taub, M.D., for reaffirming the goodness of being a physician.

To Roslyn and Daniel, my mother and father, who taught me love is all there is.

To my darling daughter Lora Taub, who diligently helped me write this book.

To Editor Douglas Corcoran and Production Editor Zsuzsa Neff, for faith and patience.

To my wellness counselor, best friend and dear wife, Anneli Taub, for inspiration, nourishment and the "Garden of Eating."

To Paramahansa Yogananda and to Sathya Sai Baba.

—*Namaste*—

Other Books by the Author

Voyage to Wellness, Anaheim, CA: Wellness America, 1988.
Prescription for Life, Anaheim, CA: American Wellness Association, 1989.

Contents

Foreword

This is the best book on holistic health care that has ever been written. It is practical, easy to understand and helps you to get well. I give it my highest recommendation.

THE WELLNESS Rx gives us the tools to take responsibility for our health. In general, Americans have received too much technology, too much surgery and too much medication. Now we have a program that allows us to participate in our health care and recapture our Natural Healing Power.

As we refocus this power, THE WELLNESS Rx points out that we are spiritual beings practicing to be human, not human beings needing practice to be spiritual. Dr. Taub has given us a new healing paradigm that ranks with the top ten health advances of our century and this Soulful Medicine will lead us into a healthy 21st Century.

Jack R. Ludwick, M.D.
Assistant Clinical Professor of Surgery
Harbor/UCLA Medical Center, Torrance, California

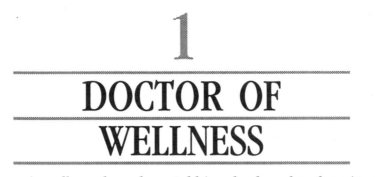

1

DOCTOR OF WELLNESS

Re-examine all you have been told in school or church or in any book, and dismiss whatever insults your soul.

—*Walt Whitman,* Leaves of Grass

The Wellness Rx introduces you to an Angel of Healing, establishes the principles of Soulful Medicine, and teaches you a strategy to cultivate your radiant energy and vital health.

The Wellness Rx will allow you to overcome stress and increase your resistance and immunity to disease. Stress is the major virus of the age and affects virtually every man, woman, and child in America. Stress is ruining health, happiness, and lives—physical stress from addictions, lack of exercise, junk food, and pollution; mental stress from worry, fear, and insecurity; and spiritual stress from isolation, each person from another and from his or her own true self. In this age of stress, your health is primarily determined by personal responsibility, self-value, and reverence for life.

EVERYONE CAN BENEFIT

To every reader who is sick and tired of being sick and tired, this book provides practical lessons and tools for cultivating healing energy and bountiful health.

If you are already healthy and well, you will benefit from the opportunity this book provides to delve deeper into the very nature of your vitality. It will support and reaffirm what you are already doing to control your health destiny and help you examine any lingering false assumptions about illness.

To those who are living with arthritis, anxiety, depression, obesity, backache, chronic fatigue, colitis, irritable bowel syndrome, insomnia, migraine, alcoholism or nicotine addiction, this book reveals the answers to

1

three essential questions that you must ask yourself to regain control of your health destiny:

- What are the *real* roots of my problem?
- What can I do in general to contribute to my recovery?
- What can I do specifically that physicians, medicine, and surgery cannot?

Because the techniques revealed in this book are as spiritual as they are scientific, they are optimal approaches to summoning the inner natural resources that reside in every person. These are the resources that have the power to restore health where health has withered and magnify health where health already dwells.

The Wellness Rx is formulated to enable you to experience and express health and wellness in all its physical, mental, and spiritual attributes. You will become aware of the fact that your life has meaning and purpose. Nobel Laureate physicist David Bohm has pointed out that even the very atoms of a human being are invested with meaning and purpose.

Your meaning and purpose are absolutely as important as the particles and electrical charges that scientists spend all their time measuring. You are on a spiritual pilgrimage back to the heart of God. Physicist Albert Einstein once commented that God was not just rolling dice and gambling when he created the universe. The good doctor also stated that the life of the individual has meaning and purpose only insofar as it aids in making the life of every other living thing nobler and more beautiful. I believe that my meaning and purpose in life are to teach my patients that God is present everywhere and in every living thing.

THREE REASONS TO QUESTION YOUR DOCTOR

Scientists, of course, say that meaning and purpose are interesting and nice but not scientific and therefore not valid. Medical scientists in particular are trained to think this way, but there are major reasons to question their attitudes:

1. According to a recent study in the *New England Journal of Medicine,* one out of every three sick or hurting Americans is using alternatives to scientific medicine. These patients reportedly even

paid $10 billion out of their own pockets without reimbursement by insurance companies. Most surprising was the fact that 83 percent of those turning to alternative, less scientific therapies, first sought treatment for the same condition from their scientific medical doctor.

2. Most of the world's physicians outside England, Canada, and the United States believe that there is a natural and spiritual aspect to health and healing and make efforts to balance an inner life force in their patients.

3. According to another report in the *New England Journal of Medicine*, traditional scientific health care may create as much disease as it cures. Dr. Franz Inglefinger wrote an editorial commenting that medical science cures about 10 percent of illness and disease. He also pointed out that medical science was *responsible* for causing about 10 percent of our illnesses, due to the side effects of medication and the unintended complications of surgery.

Obviously, it is important to take advantage of the best that medical science has to offer, but it is equally important for you to take personal responsibility to do whatever is necessary to help with your own healing process. *Your health is much too important to be unscientific about, but it is also much too important to just leave up to science.*

President Clinton is correct: the medical system is broken. Americans have overwhelmed technology and become the most overweight, atherosclerotic, ulcer-ridden, arthritic, hypertensive, cancer, coronary, and stroke-prone population in the entire world.

Near-miracles of technology have turned against Americans, who have become the most overmedicated, overradiated, oversurgerized people in recorded history. America spends more to repair illness and disease than virtually all the other nations of the world produce in total each year— *added together!*

Our entire planet is in deep trouble. Splitting the atom has led to a hoard of weapons that can destroy the earth a thousand times. Misdirected science has also led to the destruction of the ozone, the changing of the weather, the acidification of the rain, the polluting of the air, the shifting of the tides, the decimation of the forests, the poisoning of the food chain, and the wiping out of a species of life every twenty minutes. Simply stated, technology without God has created more limits than breakthroughs for humankind.

Technology, with God, is limitless.

I know from my three decades of experience with patients that your doctor will benefit immeasurably when you become actively involved in your own healing process, invested with hope and determination. The Wellness Rx is based on a new and dynamic patient–doctor relationship that brings to the treatment process the best in *both* parties. I feel honored to be a physician. I feel especially honored to be your Doctor of Wellness.

POWERFUL OUTLOOKS

Two unforgettable phases in my profession as a physician have most defined the vision of health care that I present in this book. The first phase encompasses the extensive work and effort I devoted to caring for children during my first fifteen years specializing in the practice of pediatrics. The first breath of life and the smile that a newborn shares with all present and the imagination and courage that a child with leukemia musters despite the fearful experience of his or her illness taught me a different language than my medical textbooks and professional journals.

I learned that much of our capacity to live healthfully as adults depends on our ability to become fluent once again in the childlike language of imagination, courage, and fearlessness. Thousands of children taught me to understand how our health would benefit if we were a bit more childlike.

I truly learned the full importance and meaning of this lesson in the second phase of my career, during the last fifteen years while practicing family medicine and treating individuals of all ages. Many of my patients were remarkable—not so much for the nature of their illnesses, but rather for the magnitude and sincerity of their will to become well. With courage and curiosity, often like that of a child, thousands of individuals have taken brand-new steps toward caring for their own health by learning to live by the practices I describe in this book. I tell their stories in this book, chronicling the experiences of those who learned how to overcome their obesity; break the stranglehold of their nicotine addiction; the grip of their depression, asthma, migraine, back pain, or insomnia; and much more.

Thousands of my patients courageously let go of old habits and attitudes and "grew" new ones. They learned to harness their energy and imagination in the pursuit of radiant health, and their triumphs over illness and disease reminded me of the very qualities of trust and faith that children first taught me were so central to healing.

You will read stories of common folk who were willing to become like spiritual warriors to take control of their own health destiny—"Warriors of Wellness." These patients fought not only disease itself but the perceptions and beliefs—or lack of beliefs—that were limiting their ability to be well. I tell stories of triumphant health that illustrate the most important lessons of this book. The patients' encounters with illness and their willingness to enlist their own resources to get well are touching examples of the importance of faith, hope, and love in the healing process.

In this book, healing actions, attitudes, and images are embodied in specific and practical behaviors that will serve to ignite your own body's natural healing resources. You will be introduced to seven simple steps that when followed for just seven days will generate the necessary energy to ignite the healing power of the soul. Simple guidelines for nutrition, exercise, and meditation are described in a manner that puts each of these important factors into the context of soulful health. Easy-to-follow techniques are described in detail to bring health-inducing awareness and purpose into ordinary activities of eating, walking, and sleeping. You will learn an assortment of ways to make your daily life more meaningful and more soulful, without necessarily going out of your way to do so. You will even find almost forty nourishing and nurturing recipes that transform a regular kitchen into a veritable "Garden of Eating."

Readers wishing to go beyond treatment, seeking reason and meaning for the illnesses they endure, can explore the conceptual terrain of current medical thought described throughout the book. It is here that the biases and misperceptions of modern health care are described and the spiritual and psychological solutions are explained. Covering this terrain takes the reader all the way back to the formations of modern medical science in the period known as the Enlightenment—the historical period in which science literally lost its soul.

Finally, it is important to note that because of fear of the unfamiliar, some critics may not understand the major medical and spiritual lessons of this book—particularly the notion that it is possible to take more control of your own health destiny than we ever imagined possible. When stripped of its proper and responsible context, this proven principle of self-determination lends itself to the extreme interpretation that "if I am sick then it must be my fault." This critique misrepresents the issue as well as the efforts of the many responsible and respected physicians who are no longer willing to deny the powerful role played by a patient's attitudes, emotions, behaviors, and beliefs.

Such distortions about common-sense truths of healing are perhaps due to the lack of training that physicians receive in the arena of human emotions, relations, and faith. Confronting a patient's deepest hopes, aspirations, and faith in the face of serious disease strikes alarm in many very good doctors. It is easier to dismiss the healing effects of faith and hope than it is to understand them or explain them scientifically.

At this point I want to emphasize that the Wellness Rx does not supplant orthodox medical care. It is, however, an important addition and an adjunct to traditional therapy and an irreplaceable component in your total health strategy. The success of the Wellness Rx does not diminish the role of your physician. It only enhances the part that you personally play in establishing and maintaining your health. Please make sure to inform your doctor about the choices and changes you are making, and do not stop any prescribed medications without consulting with your doctor. The goal of this book is not to draw you away from traditional health providers but instead to draw out of *you* the healing potential that only you can provide.

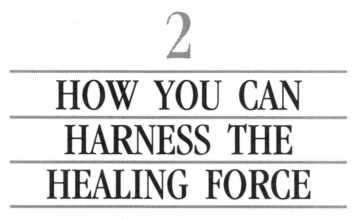

HOW YOU CAN HARNESS THE HEALING FORCE

Everyone entrusted with a mission is an angel. . . . All forces that reside in the body are angels.

—Moses Maimonides

The Healing Force is a sacred song echoing through the chambers of your heart and the deep space of your soul. It is the music that drenches your soul in joy and peace and gives strength to every cell in your body. Though we have tuned out this music with our minds, in the stillness of the soul the faint presence of the Healing Force dances. Silent no longer, from a tiny flicker to a brilliant flame, this life force renews your will to be well. Hearts are pounding with its proclamation: Awaken to wellness! Be well. Be whole.

The true narrator of this book is the Healing Force, whose mindful lessons dwell between its pages. In those who listen, that force will find expression, nourishment. In return, the Healing Force will nourish wellness within you. Above all, the Healing Force will nurture your soul, leading you on an inward path back to that source of all wellness. As the world around you struggles in turmoil, oceans of peace and calm perception linger within.

We recognize disease as our worst enemy, and yet we forget the source in every person that can overtake disease. That source is the Healing Force. It is the healing hand of the soul.

The Healing Force is like an eternal flame, burning dimly in the shadows of souls who have forgotten its soothing light. Because its hushed voice has been ignored, Americans have become the most overweight, atherosclerotic, hypertensive, diabetic, ulcer-ridden, arthritic, coronary, cancer, and stroke-prone people on this planet. Instead of fanning the flame of this awesome natural force, Americans have turned in droves to medication, surgery, and radiation. And still, within us all this time has been the patient, ever-burning, ever-soothing Healing Force.

The world is not a trivial detail, no mere accident or product of chance. God did not gamble at creation. The meaning of our presence in this magnificent universe radiates from the flickering flame of the Healing Force, the meaning that comes from within and expands outward, connecting all souls.

The meaning of this book is to raise your consciousness to embrace that long-forgotten source of healing within you.

Scientists have struggled for centuries to understand the process of healing. The Healing Force has beguiled many. Still they search in the wrong places, ask the wrong questions. For what they seek to understand is incomprehensible within the framework of the limited mind of science.

How can we comprehend logically or rationally that which is so small yet utterly infinite? How can we grasp that which exists in the minuscule atom yet encompasses the entire universe, all history, present and future? How can we make rational, scientific sense of the fact that everything— light, matter, every living and nonliving thing—is energy? Energy hurtling through time and space. Just like the soul of a human being, on a journey, back home.

Human life springs forth from energy. An explosive tiny point of light. Light becomes energy and matter. All of it in motion, moving, swirling through space.

In the beginning, there *was* light. Everything was created from that small spark of energy. Scientists are now beginning to understand this. Still incomprehensible, however, is the truth that the light that was present in the beginning is present still and will cast its brightness throughout eternity.

So much energy is beyond our mortal control but not beyond universal balance. The planets balance the sun, day balances night, dark balances light, water balances earth. Mortal minds have steadily learned to disrupt this balance. Toxic pollution chips away at the earth's protective force field. And when energy is not balanced, not integrated—when energy loses its integrity—it reaches the point of dis-integration. Isn't this precisely the effect of a nuclear bomb?

Life is more than the biological process of ever-replicating DNA. Human beings are more than mere biological organisms. There are layers to our existence. We are physical beings, individuals, yes. But we are more than that. The substance and meaning of our physical selves come from a more elusive, spiritual level of human existence. In our daily lives we are separate individuals. At this spiritual level, however, we share a connectedness not visible to the eye but felt in the calmness of mind and stillness of soul. There you experience the perfect radiant energy that is your essence. That essence is the inner flame of the Healing Force.

Life is a journey back to the perfect source of infinite energy from which we are born. The wisdom of all great religions teaches us that there is another life, a peace, a refuge in our hearts, that abides within us. Along the path back to that place we have swerved, losing sight of that tiny spark of light from which the world ascended. Prophets, sages, rainbows, miracles, and even a Son have been sent to remind us to love our bodies as sacred castles, to love the planet as the Divine Mother of all Nature, and to love our neighbors as we would be loved. Somewhere along the vast journey we have forgotten.

The Healing Force is the reminder. It is the power within you that can heal any disease. It is the nourishment of souls and the peace that can heal any heart. And there are so many hearts to heal.

In a world out of balance, disintegration manifests itself in the form of disease. In a world without balance, ill is the equivalent of I Lack Love.

The stress, worry, and anguish that threaten to shake up the calmness, happiness, peace, and health in our lives have suppressed the flow of the Healing Force. But this force is infinitely responsive. The smallest of gestures, the seemingly smallest acts of kindness and love, stoke up its flame. In this book you will learn strategies to remove the physical, mental and emotional debris that obstruct the flow of the Healing Force. It won't take drugs. It won't take surgery or radiation.

It requires energy. It requires love. *A lot of love.* And it requires meaning.

It also requires a new kind of medicine, a medicine with an expansive and inspiring mission, message, and goal. The mission is to create an awareness that your health is primarily determined by personal responsibility, self-love, and reverence for life. The message is that laughter, faith, hope, forgiveness, and love are the most powerful healers of all. The goal is to promote a world of wellness. This is the soul of science.

You have been reacquainted with the eternal patience and infinite joy of the Healing Force. Keep reading. Health and happiness are at hand.

YOUR MIRACLE OF ENERGY

The realm of the physical world, which includes all matter from the largest planet to the comparatively small human body and the tiniest cell, is the "laboratory" in which the scientist works. This is the terrain of the observable, made up of "stuff" that can be both seen and known. The realm of the spiritual, that subtle inner space in which the soul dwells, is the "laboratory" of sages and saints of all religions. Unlike the physical world, which constantly reveals itself beneath the scientist's watchful eye, the universe of the soul can be unfolded only through an entirely different science that encompasses love, compassion, consciousness, meaning, and purpose. The healing attitudes and practices you will learn about in this book bring together the knowledge of the scientists and the wisdom of the sages.

The Wellness Rx is an alternative, thoroughly responsible yet essentially soulful approach to healing and health. Given the opportunity to expand their knowledge about treatment options, thousands of my patients have reversed stress, anxiety, panic disorder, depression, and insomnia; thousands have shed excess weight, broken the shackles of nicotine and alcohol, and overcome the pain and suffering associated with heart disease, hypertension, cancer, colitis, irritable bowel syndrome, peptic ulcers, migraine, chronic fatigue, and backache. This book collects and systematizes the routine of physical, mental, and soulful practices used by patients I have cared for all over the world. Wherever you live, you will find that becoming an active participant in your own healing process has an extraordinary positive effect.

Music to the Soul

Your body is more than flesh and bones. It is a system of vital energy. If you were to take a look at any body cell under an electron microscope, you would see the tiny cell illuminating and pulsating and throbbing at rates actually beyond our vision and imagination. Every single cell in your body vibrates with electric and chemical energy. Different cells from different regions and organs of the body vibrate at different rates. An organ, your liver for example, is composed of trillions of similar cells oscillating at the same rate. A spleen cell vibrates at a different rate. An ovary cell vibrates at a still different speed.

When the cells of an organ are vibrating in harmony, the organ is healthy. For instance, when the cells of your liver are in harmony, in motion at a predetermined rate, your liver functions well and performs its physiological functions. In the proper harmonious state, the energy of your organs is in balance and contributes to the overall balance of energy in the body.

Consider a musical analogy. The sound that a violin produces is, in its essence, energy. When the violin is in tune, the sound it creates is harmonious. The strings vibrate with perfect timing, each note resonates perfectly, and the melody is clear. When just one string of the violin is just a hair out of tune, the sound energy that the instrument generates is out of harmony, out of balance.

A Glorious Composition

On a grander scale, think of that violin as part of an orchestra. When each instrument is in tune and playing on key, the orchestra creates perfection. The sound energy the orchestra produces is balanced and harmonious. If in that orchestra, however, the violin is out of tune, the system of energy that is the symphony is thrown off center, out of balance. Instead of a symphony, what we hear is cacophony, dissonance created by a poorly tuned instrument.

A similar dissonance occurs in the body when the energy of your cells or your organs is out of balance. When your body is ill, whether it be hepatitis, infectious mononucleosis, diabetes, cancer, hypertension, peptic ulcer, asthma, sinusitis, lupus erythematosus, pneumonia, sciatica, etc., etc., it just means your energy is out of sync. When the body is conceived as energy and health is perceived as the harmonious flow of energy in the body, it is easy to make the mental jump to think of disease as an energy imbalance in the body. Efforts to restore health, therefore, must logically be efforts to restore balance to the body's energy. Unfortunately, medicine, radiation, and surgery rarely restore balance and are more like Band-Aids® dealing with symptoms, not causes.

What I have described is a fairly straightforward physiological process. The roots of our understanding of energy were established by Albert Einstein, who dramatically shaped modern scientific understanding. Einstein discovered that energy is equivalent to mass multiplied by the speed of light squared ($E = mc^2$). Mass means *everything,* and it is always composed of atoms, which contain electrons and protons that carry negative and positive electrical charges and are merely nodes of energy oscillating at lightning speeds. Einstein's formula explains in shorthand that mass and energy are interchangeable. One is the other. *Everything is energy.*

The Wisdom of the Body

The human body is energy. There is also a distinctive aspect of energy underlying the physiological processes of the human body, a super-energy. This super-energy is characterized by *meaning* and *purpose.* Our bodies are orchestrated by this inner wisdom, a super-energy that informs all cellular activity in the body and infuses us with meaning and purpose. "Soulful Medicine" explores how meaning and purpose are as much a part of our energy as are the electrical charges measured on an electrocardiogram or found in a brain wave. It is sufficient at this point for you to just think more expansively about energy and understand that the meaning and purpose of your life surge through every cell of every organ, muscle, bone, artery, vein, and capillary along with the electrical charges of your energy.

What determines the rate of your liver cell's vibration as compared with a cell in the lining of your lung? What is the wisdom that regulates the communication between your cells and organs to create the perfect energy system that is your whole body?

Let's ask the question in a different way, recalling the image of the orchestra. Like the conductor, who directs and communicates with the players of the many instruments in an orchestra, is there a mechanism that conducts the energy of the multitude of elements and organs that constitute the body? Is there a force that orchestrates this magnificent symphony of energy that is the human body?

The Healing Force. An Angel with a singular mission—your safe return home. You are a soul on a pilgrimage, hurtling through time and space just like stardust, until you return to the heart of God.

To the extent that you care for your body as a temple for your soul and have forgiveness and love in your heart, your journey home will be filled with bliss. If you neglect your temple or lack forgiveness and love, your journey may become troublesome. ILL may become equivalent to **I Lack Love.**

You are a system of energy. You are a spiritual being practicing to be human, not a human being practicing to be spiritual. The Healing Force is forever whispering to you: "grow . . . grow . . ."

Your body, as a system of energy, expands outward from your flesh and intertwines with all other patterns and flows of energy in the world. The boundaries between your body and the rest of the universe—the borderline between your arm, for example, and the air that surrounds it—is not a physical boundary, only a boundary of your perception.

Dr. Deepak Chopra challenges his patients to push at the edges of their perception and see themselves as connected to the energy patterns uniting the cosmos. He likens people to candles or stars, concentrated energy inextricably linked to the infinite field of energy that gives birth to and sustains human life.

The energy of your body is inextricably woven into the fabric of the universe. But the task of unraveling this fabric to see the patterns of threads that weave your life together through space and time is a difficult one. Your self-perceptions are shaped by a strong sense of individualism and the belief that you are essentially separate from others and the world that surrounds you. This individualism, rooted in your demanding ego, dulls your sense of connectedness to others and to the origins of the world you live in.

You are a thread in the very fabric of all life. What touches others touches you. What touches you touches others. See yourself as a star in a vast constellation of souls swirling around you—your mother, your children, your friends, your neighbors, your coworkers, your community, your nation, and the world. You are the sun. How can you help bring balance to your star and the souls in your constellation? *This is your purpose and mission.*

THE BRIDGE TO WELLNESS

Throughout history, philosophers, theologians, and physicians have compared our lives to stars, those brilliant masses of energy and light that have guided travelers and enchanted poets. Within every individual is the source of the entire universe, and it is this that infuses us with meaning.

The heart of the universe dwells in the heart of all human beings. Unfortunately, this truth has become concealed beneath the layers of personality, ego, and consciousness that constitute the "individual" you know yourself to be. Nonetheless, your individualized life, your unique personality, is rooted in one common ground, an inexhaustible storehouse of energy that breathes life into you.

The Healing Force nurtures the harmony of your body and derives its energy from the sacred universal storehouse of energy. This universal energy is the very same source that creates a towering oak from a minuscule acorn; fashions trillions of snowflakes, no two patterns alike; coordinates the celestial dance of the seasons; and holds heaven and earth in balance. This universal energy is the seed, the root, the flower of all living things. How powerful is this source of energy within the human body? How magnificent is its presence? How bright is this star? Hidden within each of us, according to one expert, in each gram of flesh, is enough energy to run the city of Chicago for forty-eight hours!

Concentrated in the powerful energy storehouse that is your body, the Healing Force responds to a wisdom far superior to that derived from the intellect. Indeed, often it is our intellect that stands in the way of the "circuitry" that conducts the flow of the Healing Force throughout the body. It is your thoughts and your ideas about life, health, love, and meaning that cast mental shadows over the would-be brilliant light the Healing Force casts throughout your body.

The Wellness Rx will teach you how to calm energy-depleting thoughts and to replace them with energy-inspiring actions and beliefs. This process of cultivating inner wisdom, not of the intellect but of the soul, is also explored throughout this book. This wisdom or force with the power to protect you from every illness and disease is rooted in the source of all souls. This *universal* wisdom nourishes your sense of connectedness, a sense that may have been lost in the process of asserting who you have been led to think you are.

You experience illness and disease when your energy is no longer in balance, and therefore the Wellness Rx is formulated to bring physical, psychological, and spiritual balance back to your magnificent energy system.

The great ailment of the twentieth century is the spiritual vacuum we live in, but words spoken centuries ago by the Greek philosopher Epicurus continue to shine a beacon of hope: "It is never too early or too late to care for the well-being of the soul."

The Wellness Rx consists of seven promises to be kept for seven days. Its path leads to the heart of the relationship between the pain in your body, the worry in your mind, and the commotion in your soul.

Modern scientists and physicians who also think expansively about our energy refer to the body's healing capacities as a force known as *homeostasis*. Homeostasis describes the body's self-regulating processes by which equilibrium and proper functioning are preserved and maintained. Dr. Dean Ornish and others write about "physical, emotional, and spiritual homeostasis"—a redefinition that opens up new ways of approaching and treating illness.

Wellness is the wholly balanced state in which the energy of body, mind, and soul are so finely attuned to each other that distinctions between them dissolve and the ultimate source of our strength emerges—the Healing Force. In the following chapters you will learn how to enhance and direct the natural healing processes already occurring in your body. The Wellness Rx helps you to unfold your natural-healing state more fully from within, to experience a life of dynamic health and energy.

Every body—every ill, stressed, diseased, and depressed body—has the potential to be well. The first step on the bridge to wellness must be a firm belief that health is not given to you by others, nor does it enter you from outside your body. Your health is sacred and emerges from deep within you at your very core. To realize and experience this phenomenon may require some of the fearlessness of an infant learning to walk for the first time. The next chapter will guide you through this physical, emotional, and spiritual challenge. You will learn that fostering this type of fearlessness requires only a willingness to think differently about your body, your health, and your beliefs.

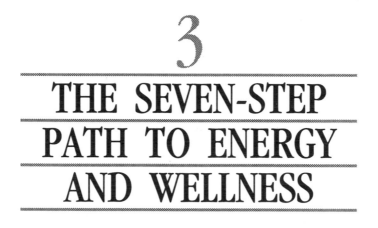

THE SEVEN-STEP PATH TO ENERGY AND WELLNESS

You will read nothing of shots or pills in these pages describing the Wellness Rx: seven promises followed for seven days to unleash the power of your Healing Force. Nothing about expensive exams or painful procedures. Indeed, the Wellness Rx resembles none of the prescriptions any physician has ever given you. Without needles, pills, or negative side effects, the Wellness Rx achieves three goals:

- It dissolves the mental, physical, and emotional obstacles hindering the flow of energy in your body.
- It stimulates your immunity and increases resistance to disease.
- It shields you from the harmful effects of stress.

A WELLNESS RX FOR LESS STRESS

Stress is so pronounced in our lives that we have invented a new term just to describe that state of pressure: "stressed-out." The description accurately conveys the typical physiological, mental, and spiritual response to stress with which most of us wish we were less familiar. Consistently confronted with stress, we constantly pour tremendous amounts of energy into the source of the stress. We typically greet a stressful event or situation with worry, anger, anxiety, and fear. Even when we attempt to ignore something stressful we tend to wrap ourselves up in figuring out ways to keep our minds off "it," thinking up strategies to avoid "it," whether "it" is a person, a thing, a day, or a time.

"Stressed-out" means that your energy literally *is* pouring outward in a chaos of directions, heading everywhere but within, where it is most

17

needed. The energy in the form of worry, anger, fear, or anxiety you project outward into stressful situations is precious energy that would otherwise be focused inward to maintain balance between your body, mind, and soul. And since disease emerges from an imbalance of energy, it is essential that you have a strategy for keeping your energy in balance—this is the promise of *The Wellness Rx:*

- to bolster your immune system,
- to redirect your energy soulward,
- to stimulate your Healing Force.

Once this process begins, your own sense of hardiness and empowerment increases resistance to the stressful factors that can cause disease. When you then focus your energy soulward, you start to literally feel a new sense of health, a total health, which can shatter the chains of illness and disease, both mental and physical.

EXPERIENCE BOUNDLESS HEALING

Let's put the process of healing in perspective. The dynamic of homeostasis is already naturally and unceasingly happening in your body. Your Healing Force is always at work, whether you command it or not. However, if you learn to tap into this process and actually enhance it, you can take greater control of the factors that impede its flow. The Wellness Rx helps to unleash a boundless source of healing and protection for you. Instead of being "stressed-out," you become physically strengthened, mentally empowered, and ultimately embraced by the strong and protective arms of your soul.

Think of this seven-day and seven-promise Wellness Rx for treatment and prevention as a spiritual timeout. It is a week lived according to seven promises that you make to yourself. The Wellness Rx fosters the unobstructed flow of your healing energy to where your energy system is out of balance and soulward to promote the enormous healing potential within you. The seven personal promises to be followed for seven days are simple and easy to follow, yet the Wellness Rx is a proven potent agent for significant improvement and change. The promises involve addictions, nutrition, love, exercise, ethics, meditation, and forgiveness.

These promises that you make to yourself and pledge in writing to follow are more important and have more impact on your health than any promise you can make to any physician. The key to the clinical effectiveness of the Wellness Rx, however, is that each and every promise must be kept so that the Rx is not taken in vain but with deepening awareness, sincerity, and a sense of sacredness.

Why does the Wellness Rx take seven days? Why does it consist of seven promises? Because real healing, healing through the soul, happens that way. Healing is a process, not an event, and must be cultivated from within you, not from without.

So follow now as we build a bridge to wellness together, with seven pillars of support, and take a seven-day journey to the other side.

I strongly urge you to read this portion of the book in its entirety to familiarize yourself with all seven components of the Wellness Rx. Then in Chapter Eleven I will ask you to sign your own Wellness Rx. Signing *your* name to the Wellness Rx will carry the weight of your own natural *inner* physician and set the healing process in motion.

For now, the only promise that you must make is that you will not skip over any chapters that don't seem to interest you at first. For example, some patients have initially shied away from the exercise portion. Others are willing to read everything but the food recommendations. Still others resist the ideas about love and forgiveness. You must read each section, even the ones that ask you to do something you may not want to—like cutting back on caffeine or forgiving a friend who may have wronged you. In fact, it might help to read the particular problematic section twice, because where you find a source of resistance, you may also uncover a source of healing. Remember this is a *prescription:* you cannot choose to just take some of the ingredients and not others. It just doesn't work that way.

WHO NEEDS THE WELLNESS RX?

In my medical experience, the patients who have benefited most dramatically from the increased flow of energy stimulated by the Wellness Rx have been those with angina, atherosclerosis, coronary artery disease, hypertension, asthma, allergies, arthritis, cancer, backache, colitis, irritable bowel syndrome, peptic ulcer, gall bladder disease, diverticulitis, diabetes, sinusitis, frequent upper-respiratory-tract infections, migraine and tension headaches, chronic fatigue syndrome, mitral valve prolapse, TMJ syndrome, premenstrual stress syndrome, osteoporosis, anxiety, depression, insomnia, panic disorder, alcoholism, tobacco and drug addiction.

Of course, not every one of my patients with these particular symptoms or conditions was "cured." However, one or more or all of the following occurred:

- The progress of the disease was significantly slowed.
- The physical or mental suffering related to the disease was decreased.
- The disease was reversed and tissues and organs were repaired.

The Wellness Rx works from the inside out: it addresses physical imbalance, psychological stress, and the soul aches and longings that underlie most illness and disease. By bolstering the healing system already present in your body, the Wellness Rx can enhance the effect of external interventions like medications or surgery and in some instances eliminate the need for them altogether.

Honoring the integrity of your own Healing Force, the Wellness Rx fosters lasting healing and protection. Responding to the soul call that illness sends out, the Wellness Rx may not always lead to the elimination of physical symptoms, but it will alleviate the soul sickness that is larger than the physical illness itself. Soul sickness is larger than physical symptoms because whereas symptoms are restricted to the individual's body, the soul is connected to all life, all forms of energy, and to the very soul of God.

EXERCISE 1—YOUR CURRENT HEALTH PROFILE

The following two exercises will help you identify old attitudes about illness and health and cultivate a new understanding of wellness. Everything that I have previously explained in this book will be much more comprehensible when you have pulled the weeds of your mental images about illness. It is particularly important that you complete these exercises before beginning the next part of the book, which addresses your relationship with physicians.

The basic conceptual principles underlying this book are worth summarizing here for your convenience and further reflection:

- Everything is energy.
- Health is the harmonious balance of energy in the body, mind, and soul.
- Disease is the breakdown of harmony in your energy.

- Every illness is anchored in your thoughts.
- If your thoughts can invite illness, they can also open the gateway to wellness, joy, and reverence for life.
- Adding just one joyful, peaceful thought to your repertoire of mental images can melt the misperceptions of illness that seem frozen into the unconscious.
- If you change your mind, you change your world.

This exercise will help you locate the seeds of illness-inviting thoughts embedded in your mental outlook. Answer the following questions with honesty and without judging yourself or anyone else. However you respond, do not let guilt or embarrassment be a part of your response. I am simply asking you to do the creative diagnostic work of identifying the sources of your perception of illness and health. Like the physician's diagnosis, this must be done openly and honestly. Write down your answers and think of this as the first entry in your "travel diary" on your journey toward wellness.

- How often are you sick? Frequently? Occasionally? Rarely? According to your perception, what would you define as frequent, occasional, or rare (how many days out of a month or year)?

- Would you characterize yourself as generally healthy or generally unhealthy?

- How many times a year do you see a physician for other than an annual checkup?

- When you count up how many days you are ill in a typical month and multiply that number by twelve, how many days are you ill during the whole year? More than you expected? Less?

- How many days have you missed this year due to illness or medical appointments?

- Were you sick often as a child? What kinds of illnesses did you have? Were these similar to the illnesses you experience as an adult?

- Does it seem like you experience more illness now than you did when you were a child? Explain please.

- What did you learn as a child about health, from your parents or other relatives, friends, school, or other sources of information?

- Were your parents generally healthy when you were a child? What kinds of illnesses did they encounter? Are any of their illnesses similar to those you experience?

- Do you see any resemblances between your parents' outlook on health and your own? Explain please.

- In general, do you feel optimistic about your health? Are you afraid of illness? Or do you feel like you are at least somewhat in control of your health destiny? Explain please.

Based on this exercise, give yourself a diagnosis about the nature of your outlook on illness. Don't get bogged down in medical terminology or clinical discourse; think generally and creatively about the history of your health and perceptions about illness. From the list below, choose a word or two that best characterize the essence of your current awareness about your personal health and well-being:

comfortable	uncomfortable
optimistic	skeptical
positive	negative
empowered	powerless
hopeful	hopeless

encouraged   frustrated
enthusiastic   anxious
proud   concerned
secure   worried
pleased   upset

If you chose words in the left column, you are already "well" on the path to wellness. If the words that characterize your outlook on illness belong to the column at the right, review your responses to the questions above and answer the following questions:

- Did your illness outlook originate while you were a toddler, while you were in elementary school, in adolescence, or adulthood? (If you don't think you know the answer, close your eyes and take a deep breath. Then ask yourself: "If I did know the answer, what would it be?")

  Check one: Explain your answer:

  When a toddler   ❏
  In grade school ❏
  Teen years   ❏
  Adulthood   ❏

- From where did your perceptions originate? Your parents? Grandparents? Siblings? Television? Friends? Spouse? Who? (Again, if you don't think you know the answer, close your eyes for a moment and take a deep breath. Ask yourself: "If I did know who it was, it would be . . .") Explain your answer.

It is important to your health that you attempt to locate the origins of your depressed outlook. Only then can the process of real healing begin. If you have identified the potential sources of your perceptions toward illness, you are already progressing on this journey toward wellness, and much of the hardest work is done.

If you selected a combination of words from both columns, take a look at your responses and try to discern where your mix of beliefs originates.

- How important are these beliefs to you? How attached to them do you feel?

- Is it possible that you no longer believe these things about your health to be true?

Write down any thoughts you have in response to the series of questions in this exercise. When you have done this, you will be able to enhance your affirming attitudes and neutralize the ones that invite illness.

EXERCISE 2—CULTIVATE A MENTAL GARDEN OF WELLNESS

Your feelings, beliefs, and expectations exercise tremendous influence over your biochemical disease-repressing and disease-repairing mechanisms. Your perceptions have the further power to *enhearten* or *encumber* the current of your body's healing energy. This vital energy has the boundless strength to keep disease at bay and to suppress the spread of disease once it emerges. Your thoughts about illness can be self-defeating ("illness is inevitable," "genes are destiny," "I just have to learn to live with disease"), or they can be self-motivating ("genes do not have the final word," "I can learn to live without disease," "the most powerful healer is within me"). This exercise is designed to help neutralize illness-inviting thoughts while cultivating those that encourage and enliven the vitality of your healing force.

Because every thought triggers a biochemical response, affirming thoughts ignite health-affirming responses. Affirmations uttered with earnestness and belief are like seeds that you can plant in the garden of your mind. Nourished with the light of your soul, these seeds will blossom into the flowers of a new outlook on health and inner wellness. In combination with the wellness-provoking steps introduced earlier in this book, affirmations are a key to dismantling the crumbling architecture of negative attitudes toward illness and mapping new wellness-oriented mental blueprints.

Yogananda describes the infinite benefits of affirmations for overcoming physical, mental, and spiritual illness: "Words saturated with sincerity, conviction, faith, and intuition are like highly explosive vibration bombs, which, when set off, shatter the rocks of difficulties and create the change desired."*

---

*Paramahansa Yogananda, *Where There Is Light*, 29.

With conviction, faith, concentration, and intuition, repeat the following affirmation. First repeat it slowly in silence, just affirming inwardly. Repeat the affirmation a second time in a soft whisper, and then a third time in your normal speaking voice. Return to a whisper, and finally affirm silently to yourself. Linger silently for a moment, with your eyes closed, listening to the hum of the words within. Throughout the day, remind yourself of the feeling of calm that accompanies heartfelt affirmation and repeat the process as often as you wish. Even uttering an affirming sentence to yourself as you work at your desk will nourish the flowers of thought now growing in your mental garden of wellness.

> *My mind is a starry garden and I am the gardener.*
> *There are no weeds of illness there,*
> *only flowers of boundless health*
> *that the perfect light of my soul inspires.*

How Wellness Can Work for You

Whether you are experiencing illness or disease, whether you are just sick and tired of being sick and tired, or whether you are fairly healthy and just want to feel "better," the basic Wellness Rx is the same: seven promises pledged in writing, to be kept for seven days. Individuals with specific problems, nicotine addiction for instance, or with chronic long-term illnesses will require added prescription ingredients and one or more prescription refills. Furthermore, individuals with life-threatening illnesses such as cancer or AIDS should incorporate these promises modified according to their circumstances as part of their daily lives forever.

Everyone—regardless of current health—should self-administer the Wellness Rx at least once a year or as often as is necessary and convenient: a week each month, a week each season, or perhaps a week during Easter and Christmastime. You may refill the Wellness Rx as often as you like. **THERE ARE NO SIDE EFFECTS.** The prescription will recharge your energy and revitalize your life; once you've experienced that boundless rejuvenation, you will never want to return to illness-inviting behaviors and beliefs again. The sevenfold Wellness Rx triggers the process of disintegrating harmful thoughts and actions and harvests in their absence mental, soulful, peaceful health. It takes seven days and seven promises to set these wheels in motion, but the underlying principles are forever.

Remember, before we move on, that the Wellness Rx is not meant to replace any traditional medical care you may currently be receiving. If you are taking prescription medication, scheduled for surgery, undergoing radiation or chemotherapy, or otherwise under the care of a doctor for a specific condition, continue with your treatment until you have properly consulted with your physician. In some situations, this Wellness Rx may be an appropriate and responsible alternative to the care you are receiving; however, that should be determined by your doctor and perhaps confirmed or disconfirmed by the second opinion of another doctor. Whatever your condition, however, by using the Wellness Rx you will create a more favorable environment for more traditional treatment to work.

Now, follow along as we construct the bridge toward wellness—seven pillars of support, seven days to journey across.

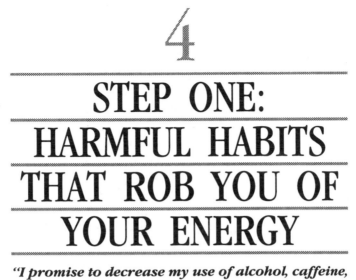

4

STEP ONE: HARMFUL HABITS THAT ROB YOU OF YOUR ENERGY

"I promise to decrease my use of alcohol, caffeine, and tobacco."

This chapter discusses the first of the seven steps of the Wellness Rx. Recall that your body is a system of energy and that all other matter is composed of energy too. Alcohol, caffeine, and tobacco are energy. As far as your body is concerned, they are foreign energy incompatible with the natural flow of your energy system. These substances disrupt the balance of your own natural life energy and place tremendous strain on the Healing Force trying to achieve and maintain harmony, or homeostasis, in your body.

The Healing Force is encumbered by the polluted energy of toxic foreign substances, which block its naturally even flow throughout the body and soul. Imagine a stream with small creeks running off in different directions, all fed by the same source of water. When the natural supply of water is healthy and fresh, water courses along the main stream and flows out freely through its creeks. Nature places rocks, boulders, trees, and shrubbery along the path of the stream, keeping the harmony of the current in check. Toss an aluminum can into the stream, a candy bar wrapper, a bag of trash, and the natural current is interrupted. When the debris piles up, the water in that area becomes polluted and may stop flowing altogether.

THREE ENERGY THIEVES—ALCOHOL, CAFFEINE, AND TOBACCO

Alcohol, caffeine, and tobacco have the same effect on the currents of energy streaming through your body. When too much of this foreign energy builds up, your body's ability to break it down and flush it out wears down. And when all of your energy is being used to remove the obstacles that foreign energy places in the path of the Healing Force, the balance in your energy system is thrown out of sync. At those moments, as you now know, the normal gatekeepers that keep illnesses at bay are no longer able to do their job. The templates of your ancestors' diseases residing in you become prematurely unleashed.

As an energy system, you are always changing. These changes are to some extent tied to your age. Have you noticed that whereas when you were in your twenties you were able to drink three beers or glasses of wine and feel nothing, now perhaps after one or two beers you may feel tired and knocked out? The reason for this change in response to foreign energy like alcohol is that your energy system has changed. Actually, alcohol-related problems are now the single biggest cause for hospitalization in the elderly—*more than cancer.*

During the week of the Wellness Rx, it would be best if you completely eliminated alcohol. If you feel you absolutely must have a drink, then limit it to only once during the week and not more than one beer, cocktail, or glass of wine. However, if you are regularly drinking fair amounts of alcohol, suffering ill effects from it, or drinking for emotional reasons, I encourage you to make an additional promise to just stop completely for an extended amount of time or forever. If you are having a problem with alcohol, it would be good for you to attend some kind of substance abuse program, such as Alcoholics Anonymous.

What better resource could you possibly ask for than AA? It integrates spirituality with science, it is nonsectarian, it is based on community support, it is free, if you can't go to them, they will come to you, and best of all, it works.

Break Your Coffee Break

If caffeine is your addiction or weakness, if you rely on coffee, tea, or diet Coke® or Pepsi® to get you through the morning and into the evening, you also need to scale back your consumption of this foreign energy. When

I ask many of my patients how much coffee they drink, their response is, "One or two." Now, I usually assume these numbers refer to cups. But for many, "one or two" refers to *pots* of coffee consumed daily!

It should be fairly clear to see that caffeine jolts your natural energy. For some it provides a "kick" or a "jump-start" in the morning, sending their energy into overdrive. For those who drink up to a pot or more a day, overdrive may seem like the natural state. In fact, some people may be so addicted to caffeine that jitters and nervousness now appear when they don't drink coffee. Wellness, however, is based on balanced energy—caffeine shakes up that balance.

Caffeine is a major cause of restlessness, anxiety, inability to concentrate, and headaches. It is a rare emergency room that doesn't see patients complaining of altered heart rhythms occurring after a coffee and caffeinated-soft-drink binge. Even one cup of coffee a day may increase the miscarriage rate in pregnant women.

For the week of the Wellness Rx, promise to drink no more than two caffeine-containing cups of coffee or tea a day and avoid caffeinated soft drinks altogether. Substitute decaffeinated coffee or tea only if you really feel you need to fill the absence. Herbal tea is the best choice—hot and steamy like coffee, it contains no caffeine.

Stop Slaughtering Yourself

No foreign energy is more destructive to your energy balance than cigarettes. You know the harm that cigarette smoking does to your lungs and your heart; you have heard the warnings from the U.S. Surgeon General. You also know what your secondhand smoke does to your children and others around you who are forced to breathe smoke-filled air. Almost 500,000 Americans die painfully and prematurely each year because of cigarettes. It's a slaughter!

What you may never have thought about before, however, is how smoking disrupts your natural energy. Seen from the perspective of energy, the obstructions smoking puts in the way of the Healing Force may lead to the instabilities of energy that cause numerous diseases of which lung cancer and bronchitis are only the most obvious. Cigarette smoking disrupts the body's energy system so drastically that it also unlocks the patterns and blueprints of asthma, allergies, heart disease, hypertension, migraine, colitis, peptic ulcers, arthritis, and much, much more. There is just no doubt that smoking disturbs the natural balance of energy in your body and consumes energy that otherwise would be spent keeping the templates of these illnesses locked away.

So for this week, if you smoke, consider making a declaration to just quit in seven days and follow the Stop Smoking Wellness Rx described in Chapter Fourteen. At the very least, however, cut your smoking in half during this week. A decrease of at least 50 percent of your usual nicotine intake is required to effect a change in your energy. This is also an excellent time to see your physician to discuss replacement therapy such as nicotine patches or gum. The bottom line is that cigarettes are incompatible with good health. So for seven days, make a significant change in your habit. Furthermore, if you are willing and ready, then set the last day of this week, day 7, as your "quit-smoking day." To help you in your efforts, Chapter Fourteen is dedicated entirely to laying out a specific approach to smoking cessation that will help you join the tens of millions of smokers who have already quit. *Remember that each cigarette you don't smoke adds seven minutes to your life.*

Great News for Smokers

More than three thousand heavily addicted smokers are quitting their habit each day. These ex-smokers made up their minds not to die or harm their loved ones. These addicts are being touched by the Healing Force.

Secondhand smoke is the third most common cause of preventable *deaths* in the United States! Children living in households where parents smoke have a significantly increased risk of developing cancer. About ten million children, almost 70 percent of children under five years old, live in homes where an adult smokes.

I conducted a smoking-cessation demonstration project called "Save Our Children" in Mt. Carmel, Illinois, to encourage parents to make up their minds to quit. Seventy smoking parents signed my "Stop Smoking Wellness Rx" and promised to quit for the sake of their children. My nurses provided ongoing emotional support for six months, and Lederle Laboratories supported the demonstration by generously donating PROSTEP™ nicotine patches and technical assistance.

An incredible 95 percent of the parents quit smoking by the end of six weeks! Even more astounding was the fact that at the termination of the demonstration, almost six months after it all began, 60 percent of the parents were *still* smoke-free! This was *double* the success rate of previously reported programs.

The key to the success of this dramatic demonstration was a strategy that stimulated feelings of personal empowerment. The new and shorter Quit Smoking Wellness Rx presented in Chapter Fourteen encompasses all of the lessons learned in Mt. Carmel. *The Healing Force awaits you.*

Your Addictions Began a Long Time Ago

Addiction is an illness, and ILL is equivalent to I Lack Love. In the 1930s, the secrets of the mind were just beginning to be understood. Psycho-analysts argued fiercely and wrote passionately about their insights into the workings of the mind. They exposed our unconscious longings and strivings and challenged traditional medical science to accept the power of emotions, attitudes, and feelings. A reign of discovery was launched by these "mind pioneers," and a window was provided through which we could peer into our soul. But traditional medical science refused to look through the window and has essentially failed to provide practical assis-tance for overcoming addictions.

Alcoholics Anonymous peered into the window of the soul and began the self-help movement for overcoming addictions. The stories of the many successes generated by AA demonstrate that drowning our woes in alcohol is equivalent to yearning for the pleasure of going back home—to security and serenity, the Garden of Eden, the womb. AA meetings are usually filled with formerly active drinkers desperately puffing cigarettes and drinking coffee to satisfy their oral needs.

Oral needs? Yes—warm, fuzzy feelings that existed in infancy and remain now imprinted in the brain forever. Addicts remember and yearn for the warmness but head in the wrong direction. The path toward security is not backward but forward, and the only way home is ahead. Addicts seek comforts that existed at their beginnings, but they mix up the directions for their journey.

The kingdom of peacefulness is within us, and traditional medicine has not yet been able to provide the key to that kingdom. Instead, it has developed thick books of diagnostic codes and molecular theories. We now know that the physical aspect of addiction involves receptor sites on the surface of the cells becoming linked up to addictive substances. It is difficult, however, for molecular scientists to conceive of the notion that physical receptor sites are also *psychologically* determined. This is why the pure biomedical scientific model for treating addictions has been a failure.

The Wellness Rx adds a psycho-social-spiritual approach to address the inner pain and outer isolation that cause addicts to apply the useless Band-Aids® called alcohol, caffeine, and tobacco.

A personal spiritual vacuum creates misdirected energy that can be as explosive as the violence in our cities and as ruthless as the movies and television we view. The individual and collective human psyche does not hesitate to contaminate the environment and blow up its neighbors. Why should it hesitate to destroy its own body through addictive substances.

For many individuals, the idyllic myth of infancy is surely just a myth. The tiny baby, cooing and appearing innocent and angelic, is also a bundle of energy containing powerful drives, instinctual needs, *and a lifelong capacity to remember pleasure and pain.* The little gurgler is filled with love for his or her parents and can also experience inner pain as well as rage. How shall we picture the complexities of that soul when it leaves the crib still yearning for remembered pleasures and security while entering the arena of childhood, adolescence, and adult life? How many fail? How many fall? How many are mentally and emotionally scarred and bewildered? How many become addicts who just can't hide stress behind masks of composure the way most others do?

Twenty-five percent of babies are cut out of their mother's abdomen in a blast of surgical light instead of experiencing the warm and peaceful massage of nature's birth canal. Eighty percent of male infants are subjected to an awful pain of circumcision without anesthesia during their very first day. Seventy percent of babies find themselves sucking an artificial nipple. Fifty percent will lose their mothers to the workforce, and a similar number may never know their father.

How then can grown-up infants stem the darker nights of their soul, crying for the impossible and striving for the unattainable? What kind of compass can direct them and hold them to the true north of their maturity, their self-understanding, and their peace of mind? *The Healing Force recognizes truth as distinguished from frozen memories and is able to end one's yesterdays last night.*

DETERMINE YOUR OWN HEALTH DESTINY

During this week of the Wellness Rx you will engage in the process of cultivating healthful, soulful habits that bolster rather than sap your energy supply. If you are particularly attached to any one of these addictive and energy-depleting substances—alcohol, caffeine, tobacco—you should also avoid environments you associate with them. If you spend your lunch break in the cafeteria with coworkers who smoke, eat your lunch somewhere else or outdoors; turn your coffee break into an exercise break; don't go to bars. *Environment can be stronger than willpower.*

Remember that these desires or hungers are merely attempts to mask the real hunger of the soul. But rather than feed the soul's constant craving for love and attention, these habits only distance us further from the comforting joy of the soul, the joy that satisfies all desires. Taken together, the seven promises of the Wellness Rx dislodge illness-inviting habits by erasing the mental blueprints of these habits in your mind. In place of these weedlike habits, during this Wellness Rx new behaviors and patterns of thought that truly feed the deep longings of the soul and nourish good health are cultivated.

5

STEP TWO: SUPER HEALING FOODS

"I promise to eat only fresh fruit, whole-grain cereals with skim milk and whole-grain bread or bagels before noon; to eat red meat no more than once this week; and to limit my intake of fat, dairy products, and refined sugar."

Nutrition, nourishment, nurturance. Food is a source of all three, although you may associate food with only one or two of these ideas. You know food is nutrition. And you may think of food as nourishment. But food is also nurturance for the soul. The foods you eat either contribute to or detract from the balance and harmony of your energy system. Food affects the soul, and eating soulfully nurtures the Healing Force. For most of us, however, this concept is as foreign as tofu or tabouli. So let's spend some time on its meaning.

The nutritional guidelines for the Wellness Rx are simple to follow and will simply make you feel magnificent. The almost forty recipes in the Appendix portion of this book are delicious, diverse, and easy to prepare. They will make it easy for you to start across the bridge from sickness and tiredness to wellness and boundless energy. No more distasteful diets. No more counting calories. When you learn to think of food from the perspective of energy, when you learn how to eat soulfully, you will finally be free of all of your misperceptions about food, eating, and weight.

Some of the mental blueprints most deeply rooted in our minds are those that concern food. We eat for comfort; we eat to cure loneliness, stress, or depression. But eating a bar of chocolate, a pint of ice cream, or a bag of potato chips never solves our deep aches. Indeed, this sort of mindless eating only makes us more lonely, more depressed, more upset. Eating to forget our aches literally eats away at the harmony of the body. We do need to feed our soul aches, but we need to do so mindfully and soulfully so that we can heal rather than temporarily cover up our inner longings.

35

Think about your last meal. Was it, in fact, a meal? Or was it a donut or muffin wolfed down in the car on the way to work? Or a salad scrunched in between business meetings and errands? Was it takeout that you ate while you watched the evening news? Like most things that we do, our eating habits are basically driven by the clock. Too often we eat in a rush, on the run, or while doing something we assume is more important than eating.

EATING WITH MINDPOWER

Where was your mind during that last meal? Was it on the television images of massacre somewhere in the world? Or on a business meeting planned for the next day? Or on a conversation you had had earlier in the day that upset you or made you angry? When was the last time you ate and thought about nothing but the food you were eating and the uses to which its energy would be put? Our minds are typically in the past or the future. Rarely do we let our minds just dwell on the present, observing the moment before it lapses into the next. When we put our mind into it, eating becomes a very different experience and serves a radically different purpose.

When you stop to think about what you are eating, how you are eating it, and why, you immediately have a greater awareness of your hunger and what is required to satisfy it. Not only do you appreciate the flavor of food more, but you eat less because you recognize when you have consumed the right amount of food to provide the energy your body needs. This feeling is so much more satisfying than the one that makes you want to release the top button of your pants or lie down and nap.

Dr. Dean Ornish has built a successful program for losing weight and healing coronary artery disease around the concept of eating with aware-ness and presence of mind, precisely because when we do eat with our minds in the present we tend not to overeat. According to Dr. Ornish, when we eat with other things on our mind, in a hurry, or with distractions, we feel stuffed instead of satisfied and miss part of the pleasure of eating. Dr. Ornish's program is so wonderful because it is also based on the belief that we need to find healthful ways to feed the deep hunger of our souls, a point I will say more about toward the end of this chapter.

But the Ornish program for weight loss may be too demanding for some, with its strict no-fat requirement. While the American Heart Associa-tion and others recommend consuming no more than 30 percent of your daily calories from fat, Dr. Ornish's program requires that you eat less than 10 percent fat. This is surely a goal to strive for but may not be immediate-ly realistic for some. President and Hillary Rodham Clinton have set a personal goal of no more than 20 percent fat calories a day. My clinical experience with families of all educational and socioeconomic levels has convinced me that deriving less than 25 percent of calories from fat is a feasible goal for almost everyone. The Wellness Rx takes a gradual and moderate approach to reducing fat intake. That is not to say you should not strive for a diet of less than 10 percent fat; it just recognizes that for some the difficulty of meeting such a goal may at first undermine the effort. Striving for less fat in the diet without suffering is the goal, and staying under 25 percent fat intake will be achievable by all.

Even if we are not hungry, we tend to eat at certain times during the day that we associate with eating. That association is usually stronger than the hunger itself. The true feeling of hunger, most identified with a grumbling stomach, is the body's signal that it requires more fuel to carry out its work. Unfortunately, we tend to mistake our emotional longings for food—*merely the idea that something would taste so good right now*—for the body's signs that it is time to ingest more food energy. Just the very thought "a thick pastrami sandwich with mustard and a pickle would taste heavenly right now" is enough to make the stomach grumble, the taste buds ignite, and to send the salivary glands into overdrive. Our eating patterns including meal times and food choices have been shaped largely by television and billboard advertisements that play on the emotional hunger within us. Because their emotional hunger has already driven them to be one meal ahead, many people never give their body a chance to tell them that it needs more energy.

FOODS THAT BOOST YOUR ENERGY

The goal of this week is to learn to eat with an awareness of energy—the energy of your body and the energy that makes up the foods you eat. *Changing your diet alone is not enough; it is more important that you change your ideas about why you eat, what you eat, and when you eat.* Our patterns of eating reflect our patterns of thoughts about food, diet, and our bodies. Looking at food from the perspective of energy brings an entirely different perspective to the process of eating. You will find that the foods you eat actually taste better. And because they are high in energy and low in fats and sugars, you can eat more of them without gaining weight.

From the standpoint of energy, food gives you energy or it takes energy away from you. Food that is easily digestible and readily turned into energy that the body can use gives more energy to your system than it takes away from your system through the process of digestion. These foods give you a surplus of energy. Some foods are difficult to digest and require more of the body's energy to be converted into expendable energy. Once all of that energy has been expended in the process of digestion, the supply of energy is actually negative. It takes more energy to digest these foods than the food itself provides.

From the perspective of energy, then, if we want to increase our energy and in turn bolster the Healing Force that keeps us balanced and well, we should strive to eat mostly foods that create a surplus of energy. Foods that give more energy than they absorb contribute significantly to the overall process of maintaining the harmonious state of energy you experience as good health or wellness. I call these foods "alive."

On the other hand, foods that give to the body less energy than is required to digest them diminish our energy supply. Energy that could otherwise be spent in the process of achieving and maintaining a state of balance in the body is directed instead to the stomach and intestines where it is needed to convert food into usable energy. Unfortunately, the energy these foods provide is just a tiny fraction of the energy spent to digest them. I call this second type of food "dead."

To digest food that comes from nature, food that is alive with energy, gives you energy. To digest food that is dead drains your energy. Food that comes from the earth, food that is fresh and in its natural state, is essentially living energy. Food that is created in a factory, food that is injected with preservatives and coloring agents, then canned, frozen, dried, irradiated, processed, pulverized, refined, and dehydrated has been stripped of much of its natural energy and is essentially dead. Where on earth can one find fields of flowing white bread and potato chips under the soil? Twinkies® on trees? Flowing streams of diet cola? You get the picture.

To make this distinction more clear, lets lay it all out on the table by looking at the average American breakfast, the type of morning meal endorsed, not coincidently, by the dairy, beef, pork and egg industries.

Breakfast begins with a "fresh" glass of orange juice. The label on the carton says "100% fresh orange juice from concentrate." That is misleading. Orange juice that comes from concentrate is not fresh; orange juice that comes directly from oranges is fresh. Orange juice that has been concentrated has also been refined, pulverized, crystallized, chemicalized, and, in most cases, frozen. There is nothing "fresh" about this kind of orange juice; it is dead and low in energy. Real fresh orange juice is squeezed from oranges and served soon thereafter and is loaded with vitamin C and energy.

After you drink your concentrated orange juice, the typical breakfast includes one or two eggs cooked in some manner. Boiled, fried, or poached, any way you serve it up, an egg is dead energy. Eggs have recently received negative publicity for being loaded with cholesterol, but in addition they are essentially devoid of energy.

Next to your eggs, you might have a few slices of bacon—greasy, processed, preserved dead pig. The amount of protein this food provides is hardly worth the amount of energy your body requires to digest it, a process that takes *close to three days*.

Rounding off your typical breakfast, a glass of milk. Most of us were taught in school that you need four glasses of milk a day to keep you strong and healthy. Cow milk is wonderful nutrition—if you're a calf. Many people drink milk and have no problems, but many others cannot digest milk because they lack lactase and other natural enzymes required to digest it. Milk gives many people gas and diarrhea. At one time, it was standard for doctors to recommend to patients with ulcers that they drink milk. Now we know that milk actually aggravates ulcers. Many pediatricians, including Dr. Frank Oski, chairman of the Department of Pediatrics at the Johns Hopkins Medical School, now tell mothers not to feed their babies cow's milk. While milk is a high source of calcium commonly recommended for menopausal women especially to prevent the onset of osteoporosis, the disease is actually rare in countries such as China, where women do not drink milk and are physically active and eat green vegetables regularly. It is becoming widely believed that milk simply is not the staple of a healthy diet we once thought it was.

Even my favorite cartoon character, the young Calvin of Bill Watterson's series "Calvin and Hobbes," recently stopped to consider why humans drink cow milk. Standing with his animated stuffed tiger Hobbes, Calvin asks, "Who was the guy who first looked at a cow and said, 'I think I'll drink whatever comes out of these things when I squeeze 'em'?" And in another strip, sitting at the dinner table eating a hamburger, Calvin asks his mother, "Is hamburger meat made out of people from Hamburg?" "Of course not!" his mother tells him. "It's ground beef." Stunned, Calvin asks, "I'm eating a COW?" His mom nods, "Right." Spitting out his food and tossing the hamburger from his hands, Calvin exclaims, "I don't think I can finish this."

How to Improve Your Moods Nutritionally

How do you feel after a breakfast like the one described above? Especially if you add toast made of refined, processed, and bleached white flour? Like you are ready to get back in bed for a few more hours? The reason you may feel that way is because the typical American breakfast drains your energy by requiring tremendous amounts of energy to digest it. This would not be so important a point if it weren't for the fact that the very energy required to digest your "well-rounded" breakfast is energy that is no longer available to help burn excess fat as well as suppress potential disease.

Food has a powerful effect on your mental and emotional outlook, as well as its obvious effects on how you look. A diet that is low in fat and cholesterol and abundant in complex carbohydrates has been shown to combat depression and hostility as well as lower your risk of heart disease. The foods you eat during the Wellness Rx week are alive with energy. They will benefit you physically as well as mentally and spiritually, promoting a sense of joy and reverence for life and lifting any feelings of depression or anger you may be currently experiencing. You will not need any special cooking equipment or any fancy techniques. Indeed, the best way to eat these energy-giving foods is with the minimal amount of preparation possible. The simpler the process of preparing foods, the simpler the process of digesting it. Boiling a potato changes its energy content ("nuking" a spud in the microwave literally kills its energy), while steaming it alters its energy only slightly.

TRY ALIVE FOODS AND SAY GOODBYE TO ILL HEALTH

Gray are all your theories but green the growing tree of life.
——Goethe

Obviously Goethe was not writing about diets and nutrition and all the theories that have emerged to explain why some people lose weight and others gain weight. But it is essentially Goethe's idea that underlies the impulse of my own efforts at explaining why food affects us the way it does. The basic belief inspiring the nutrition guidelines for the Wellness Rx is that food that comes from nature, from the trees and the earth, is exactly what your own nature requires. These are foods that are bursting with "aliveness."

"Alive" foods are those that are filled with energy and vitality: fresh fruits, vegetables, nuts, whole grains and complex carbohydrates (bagels, rice, pasta, potatoes). Alive food is not food that is literally now or has been previously living, such as a cow, or chicken, or lamb. Alive food never had a mother or a face. I use the term *alive* to designate foods that are literally bursting with energy and life, like a ripe apple, fresh oatmeal, a baked potato or a juicy tomato. A hamburger, a drumstick, or a thick steak is basically dead energy, or energyless.

That is not to say that there is no room in the Wellness Rx for a piece of chicken or fish, or even a hamburger. The most important guideline to this week of sensible energy-based eating is that you treat everything with moderation—including moderation! So if you must eat meat, follow these guidelines:

- Eat chicken or fish instead of red meat; baked or broiled, not fried.

- If you do eat red meat, avoid any type of meat for seventy-two hours afterward. It takes up to three days for your body to digest it, so if you are going to eat meat, at least give your body the opportunity to digest it thoroughly and get rid of it before you challenge it with more.

- Eat chicken or fish in smaller portions rather than as the main entree. Toss it on top of a large bed of pasta, rice, or salad.

My purpose here is not to convince you to become a vegetarian, although there are many compelling reasons for a vegetarian diet. The point I am trying to make is that the amount of meat Americans consume plays a significant part in the amount of heart disease, high cholesterol, obesity, hypertension, cancer, colitis, insomnia, depression, and fatigue from which many Americans suffer.

Red meat has recently been implicated in several major scientific studies as a contributing cause of breast cancer and colon cancer. Now it is believed that red meat is a major factor in prostate cancer, the second leading cause of death in men after lung cancer. It will not surprise readers of this book that prostate cancer can lie dormant for decades without causing symptoms or death. Prostate cancer often behaves in a sleepy manner and is discovered quite by surprise in almost a third of all men over age fifty who die from unrelated causes. A study of 48,000 men determined that 300 of them had prostate cancer. The researchers were stunned to find that those with the cancer ate red meat five times a week. The study concluded that eating red meat five times a week is linked to a 250 percent increase in prostate cancer, presumably because the type of animal fat in red meat triggers the dormant cancer of the prostate.

Not only is meat dead energy, it is pumped full of hormones and antibiotics. When you eat meat, you also ingest the hormones and antibiotics injected in the cow or chicken, and this affects your energy too. A doctor at the Harvard School of Public Health was recently quoted in *Vegetarian Times* as saying, "I don't like meat much. I don't think anybody in public health can like meat anymore." And while chicken is supposed to be a healthier choice than meat, "healthier" is only relative. Some 60 to 65 percent of chickens are infected with salmonella. Cooking guidelines have been provided by the chicken industry to ensure you that if cooked properly, the salmonella is killed. So not only are you eating dead chicken, you are eating dead salmonella. What do you think the salmonella did to the energy of the chicken?

You were probably taught since you were a child that you need lots of beef to grow big and strong and healthy. That simply is not true. Have you ever considered what a cow eats to be big and strong and healthy (besides antibiotics and hormones, that is)? Grass. Green, leafy grass. Now I am not advocating a grass diet for you. But I am suggesting that for this week, seven days, you eat live foods including grains and leafy green vegetables. Food that comes from the earth and dangles from the branches of trees is alive.

If we listened to our heart half as much as we listen to our taste buds, Americans would have far fewer instances of high cholesterol and heart disease. Your taste buds have essentially been programmed to like certain tastes more than others. Your taste buds may crave the flavor of meat more than vegetables, but that craving is not natural and it can be changed. Your heart does not crave meat, because meat is high in cholesterol, saturated fat, and oxidants, all of which clog your arteries and raise the amount of cholesterol in your blood.

There is a little bit of vegetarian in all of us. Think about the vegetables and fruits you like most and just begin from there.

CLIMBING THE FOOD ENERGY LADDER

Don't think of this week as a diet. It's not. But it is a timeout for your body, your soul, and your system of energy. By freeing up your energy from the difficult and consuming process of digesting foods that are hard to break down, like meat and fat, you make more energy available to enhance homeostasis and protect you against illness. Every day that you don't eat meat you bolster the supply of energy in the storehouse that is your soul. You will, literally, have more energy. And energy is the basis of good health and reverence for life.

So what should you eat? And how much? The remainder of this chapter lays out concrete guidelines for eating during the Wellness Rx week. These guidelines should be followed in conjunction with the recipes in the "Garden of Eating" (see Appendix). If you eat only these recipes for the next week, you will not even notice the absence of meat and excess fat in your diet, for they are abundant in flavor and satisfying at the same time.

You should feel free to consult other vegetarian cookbooks as well, including *The American Vegetarian Cookbook, The Gradual Vegetarian, Eat More—Weigh Less, Simply Vegetarian!, The Enchanted Broccoli Forest, The Greens Cookbook,* the Moosewood cookbooks, and any Italian recipe book that has plenty of meatless pasta dishes.

The basic guideline is this: *eat as much fresh and alive food as you wish.* If you are eating only fresh foods from nature, lots of fruits, vegetables, grains, and pastas, you need not worry about gaining weight. The Energy Ladder chart on page 44 will help you identify which foods are alive and high in energy and which ones are low on the energy ladder.

BREAKFAST—THE AMAZING ENERGY SOURCE

Several years ago I wrote the foreword to the breakthrough nutrition book *Fit for Life,* by Harvey and Marilyn Diamond. The book presents a theory of food-combining attuned to the ways that your digestive system assimilates, stores, and uses food energy. Over the years I have encouraged my patients to follow the Diamonds' strategy, combining some foods and avoiding other combinations. Many of my patients lost or gained significant amounts of weight, according to their goals, and did so without ever feeling starved or undernourished. I lost thirty-five pounds myself and had more energy than many young children. While they loved the results, many patients worried that it was difficult and time consuming to eat in the suggested manner. One patient, a celebrated cook in the community, complained that it took too much "brainwork" and spoiled the fun and spontaneity she was used to enjoying in the kitchen. Preparing meals should be pleasurable, not a chore, and a scientific basis for nutrition is important too. So I devised a nutritional plan that retains the very best of *Fit for Life* but updates it and makes it more simple to follow.

Breakfast and Before Noon

One of the most important guidelines in the Wellness Rx is that you eat a hearty breakfast each day. Breakfasts don't have to be skimpy as long as you eat the right foods. Before noon eat any of the following in any combination:

- Fresh fruit and fruit juice, as much as you like.
- Whole-grain, low-fat cereals and oatmeal without added sugar. Use only nonfat milk.

Wellness Food Energy Ladder

Fruits

Vegetables

Pastas, rice, potatoes

Whole-grain breads & cereals

Nuts, avocados, & olive oil

Fish

Poultry

Beef, pork, lamb

Non-/low-fat dairy

Regular dairy products

Eggs

Candy & sweets (refined sugar)

- Whole-grain breads, muffins, and bagels.

Because of its high energy content, fruit is the most important ingredient in a Wellness breakfast. Remember, however, that in terms of energy, canned or frozen fruit is neither alive nor equivalent to fresh fruit, so eat fresh fruit whenever possible. Be sensible. Don't stuff yourself, but eat whatever fresh fruit you want and as often as you want until noon. For variety, blend your fruit in a blender and have a "smoothie," a natural shake loaded with fresh fruit and juice and crushed ice or nonfat yogurt for a thicker shake. Fruit gives you more energy than most foods in part because it is so packed with vitamins but also because it takes almost no energy to digest. Most fruit reaches your stomach already digested. While the typical American breakfast described previously leaves you stuffed and ready for a nap, a plateful of fruit or a tall fruit smoothie fills you up but gives you a lasting surge of energy (unlike coffee or sugar, which temporarily blasts your energy and then makes you crash).

Things don't get too much more complicated than that. If you absolutely don't feel satisfied with fruit in the morning, go for the grains and breads instead. Eat your muffins or bagels or toast with a bit of fruit spread instead of butter or cream cheese. For variety, sometimes I add a slice of tomato on my toast and sprinkle it with a dash of salt, onion powder, and pepper. Finally, if you simply aren't satisfied, use a nonstick pan or one of the nonfat sprays to fry or scramble one or two eggs without their yolks.

Lunch and Dinner

For the rest of the day, emphasize vegetables, complex carbohydrates, whole grains and more fresh fruit. Avoid flesh foods. These are the foods that most make you feel like napping because they require so much energy—three days' worth—to digest. Do your energy and motivation at work fizzle out after your lunch break? This could be related to the food you are eating for lunch. Put away the bags of potato chips and eat a baked potato instead; rather than eating a pastrami sandwich, try one filled with fresh vegetables and a thin slice of cheese (try the St. John's Special included in the "Garden of Eating"); trade in your candy bar for a bunch of grapes. Pick up bits and snacks of alive food and just "graze" throughout the day. The recipes in the "Garden of Eating" will prove to you that just because you are cutting back on flesh, fat, and sugar does not mean you have to give up flavor.

LOSE FAT, NOT HOPE

We surely were not aware that the charts of the four basic food groups presented to us by our teachers and school nurses were merely advertising efforts funded by the meat, pork, dairy, and egg industries. Yet that is a major reason why Americans are the most overweight, hypertensive, atherosclerotic people in the world. The aorta of a typical three-year-old is already accumulating unhealthy deposits of fat. We simply have been miseducated about what constitutes good eating habits.

Recently, the U.S. government introduced the new "Pyramid of Food Values" to replace the fat-laden, low-energy nutrition concepts represented by the four basic food groups. It is disheartening to note, however, that the Pyramid of Food Values was promptly withdrawn because of bitter resistance on the part of the same food industries whose livelihoods have been built upon the four-food-group philosophy.

Even more disturbing is the fact that the power of the food industry was enough to eliminate the crucial "percentage-of-fat" listing in the new food-labeling laws. One can of course simply multiply the grams of fat listed on the food label by nine and then divide that number by the total number of calories listed. But it is no wonder that the vast majority of Americans find that formula too cumbersome to deal with.

If your goal is to lose excess fat permanently, safely, and with relative ease, keep your daily fat intake below 25 percent of your daily calories—the lower the better. Unfortunately, the absence of the simple percentage-of-fat figure on food labels presents a problem for individuals not interested in using the "multiply-and-divide" formula. You can, however, calculate the grams of fat. The basis of weight loss is twofold:

- If you eat excess fat you accumulate excess fat.
- If you accumulate excess fat you need more energy to burn off the excess fat.

The optimal strategy for reducing your body fat percentage is to eat fewer fatty foods as well as increase the energy available in your body to burn fat.

There are three ways to monitor and restrict how much fat you take in:

- Calculate, multiply, and divide to stay under 25 percent daily fat intake.
- Avoid animal food, animal fat, and animal products.

- Climb to the top of the Food Energy Ladder and stay within the top five rungs.

Count Blessings, Not Calories

Counting calories is generally a waste of time as far as achieving permanent weight loss. If, on the other hand, you are trying to gain weight, counting calories, especially those from complex carbohydrates, may be helpful. People trying to lose weight, however, typically get caught up in the trauma of calorie counting and often fall into a yo-yo pattern of dieting. Not only is this pattern dangerous, the rationale for calorie counting just cannot be supported. Not all calories are the same! Five hundred calories from a plate of fresh fruit is *not equivalent* to 500 calories of a high-fat serving of meat, in which nearly 80 percent of the calories come from fat. One food is alive and the other is dead.

There are some special considerations for people who want or need to lose excess weight. I typically observe in my patients who follow the nutritional guidelines of the Wellness Rx a general trimming down. That is, patients who are five to ten pounds heavier than their optimal weight for their body size and who have a higher than ideal percentage of body fat tend to lose that fat simply by following the basic nutrition guidelines. But for those who want or need to lose more than ten pounds, consider the following.

Losing excess fat permanently requires eating foods that are low in fat and are high in energy. The simple reason is that it takes high energy to burn excess fat. You will lose the excess fat and weight if you climb the Food Energy Ladder and stay on the top five rungs. Eat less dead food and fewer foods that are high in fat. Eat less flesh, fewer eggs, less dairy, fewer refined sugars and junk foods. Eat more fruits, more vegetables, more whole-grain breads and cereals, more beans, lentils and other legumes, more rice, pasta, and potatoes. Eat food that is alive and bursting with energy.

If you stay on the top five rungs of the Food Energy Ladder, you will not feel deprived and you will not have to bother with counting calories and multiplying and dividing to determine percentage-of-fat calories. Restrict your use of oils in salads and in cooking to olive oil and canola oil, and use them *sparingly.* You don't have to be a physicist or a rocket scientist to know intuitively how to eliminate 95 percent of the fat in your diet: *restrict your intake or eliminate completely animal flesh and animal products.*

You can reasonably expect to safely, scientifically, and permanently lose one pound of excess weight per week; thus, four pounds a month. If you integrate the Wellness Rx eating guidelines into your daily practices, in the course of one year you may lose fifty pounds of excess fat. Of course, that much weight loss is only appropriate for people who are severely overweight or obese, and they should work alongside with their doctors. Regular exercise and restricting alcohol intake is crucial for consistent weight loss.

If your goal is to lose excess fat, incorporate the following guidelines into your Wellness Rx nutrition plan:

- Restrict animal fat and animal products in your diet.
- Eliminate red meat.
- Limit your intake of fish or skinless poultry to no more than twice a week.
- Climb to the top five rungs of the Food Energy Ladder with food that is fresh and alive.

NATURE'S GIFTS TO YOUR HEALTH

For the Wellness Rx week, the foods you eat will give your body energy as well as nurture the soul. Think of the foods you eat not only as nourishment for your physical body but for nurturing the hunger of the soul. But remember: the soul does not hunger for junk foods or food high in fat or sugar! Only your ego craves those things and tries hard to convince you that you *must* have a dish of ice cream or a bag of chocolate candies to feel good.

Because the soul comes from nature, it hungers for nature. Feed it naturally. Just like an infant, the soul's appetite must be fed with care and love. You will achieve your appropriate weight when you begin eating the foods that nourish and provide fuel for your body as well as nurture the soul's deeper hungers.

Nourishing and nurturing nutrition means eating not until your stomach feels "full" but in a way that is "soul-full." That is, the foods you eat and the way you prepare and eat them should be soul-filled. The Wellness Rx week will help you learn to listen to your soul instead of your stomach. When you eat for energy, eating that feeds your soul, you are less likely to overeat or to eat unhealthful foods.

In terms of energy, it is extremely important to understand that the energy of the fat contained in an olive, a nut, or an avocado is simply not equivalent to the energy of the fat in a piece of bacon. We cannot scientifically explain why the recipes of the Mediterranean are awash with olive oil but the hearts of the people living in the region are not; we cannot scientifically explain why a handful of walnuts every other day seems to lower rather than increase the rate of heart attack; we cannot scientifically explain why avocado-eating kids in California seem thinner, healthier, and more full of energy than kids in other parts of the country.

It is not only the action of fat energy that science cannot completely explain. Science cannot explain why the energy we get from the sugar in an apple or an orange is different from the sugar we get from a candy bar. Nor can science explain why the energy of mother's milk is different from the energy of artificial baby formula, even though the chemical composition of both are virtually identical. It is my belief that it is simply impractical to equate what is made in a laboratory with what comes from a tree or a bush or grows from the ground. So while it is absolutely necessary that you reduce the amount of fatty oils and refined sugars that you eat, it is also important that you understand that avocados and nuts have their place on the Food Energy Ladder. Eat these foods sparingly, no more than two avocados a week and no more than a handful of unsalted nuts two or three times a week. But know that they are certainly more alive than anything invented in a laboratory.

Nurturing nutrition entails more than simply eating foods that are alive with energy. The nurturing aspects of soulful eating have a lot to do with the spirit in which you prepare your food and eat it. Do you think of cooking as a chore? Are you likely to eat out or pop a ready-made frozen meal into the microwave just to avoid the hassles of cooking and cleaning the dishes? Perhaps when you return home from work, your energy is so drained that the last thing you look forward to is preparing a meal. Eating takeout or a frozen dinner occasionally is fine, but the reasons why you eat this way may contribute to an unhealthful pattern of thinking about food. This week you must add something else.

THE SECRET INGREDIENT THAT MAXIMIZES NUTRITION

I recently read a story about a monk who is responsible for all of the cooking at his monastery. Brother Lawrence treats cooking, not as a chore, but as a spiritual celebration. Cooking, like all activities, can be transformed into a moment for remembering the presence of spirit that surrounds us.

Cooking can be more than the mundane tasks of measuring, mixing, blending, and baking. A kitchen can be a place, like a garden or a sunny creek, where you can practice the presence of a Higher Power. In Hindu lore, Lord Krishna teaches the same thought. "The world is imprisoned in its own activity, except when actions are performed as worship of God." All work, no matter how seemingly mundane, is holy when, according to Krishna, "the heart of the worker is fixed on the Highest." By focusing on the Highest and performing his responsibilities with love, the monk pours love into every dish he bakes. Since the soul feels only love, food that nurtures the soul must be filled with love.

After graduating college, my daughter spent some time at a yoga retreat in northern California. I embraced the opportunity for her to learn a different kind of knowledge than what she had acquired at the university, to study Indian philosophy and strengthen her practice of yoga. When she telephoned me after her first week at the retreat, I was stunned to hear that she was spending five hours a day in the kitchen cooking for the fifty or so retreat guests. This was supposed to be a spiritual retreat, relaxing and rejuvenating! What was she doing toiling in the kitchen?

Strangely, her voice registered no complaints. In fact, she sounded happier and more peaceful than at any other moment I recalled in her life. I asked her if there was anything I could do, someone I could talk with, to try to get her out of the kitchen and out into the gardens, where she would at least be in the fresh air and sunshine. She immediately opposed the idea. "Why would I want to do that? I find the cooking very relaxing and the food is terrific! Everyone eats with so much joy here. The looks on their faces are so satisfying to me." This did not sound like my daughter, the one who had never showed any interest in cooking for herself, let alone a crowd of fifty.

When I visited the retreat myself the following summer, I finally understood what had transformed my daughter's attitude toward cooking so dramatically. The large kitchen at the guest retreat, it seemed, was as meditative a place as the temple. Indeed, for the people preparing the wonderful vegetarian meals the guests feasted on, cooking was a form of meditation. It was not just that they prayed while they cooked but that their cooking became a prayer itself. Cooking, like everything else at this retreat, was transformed into a way of practicing the presence of a Higher Power. Singing filled the air in the kitchen and mingled with the delightful scents of curries, cinnamon, garlic, and other spices. Eating was a pleasure not just because the food tasted so great but because the entire environment made one feel joyful, nurtured.

There is no doubt that food cooked with love and spirit tastes better than food flung into the microwave in a hurry. The energy of the cook enhances the energy of the food. Obviously this is something science cannot explain, but the wisdom of the body knows better. Have you ever noticed that the food you prepare when you are exhausted and uninterested in cooking tastes bland or flavorless? In the same way, food that you prepare enthusiastically, for a party, for example, usually turns out terrific because of the effort you put into making it. You try new recipes and old favorites to make your guests feel at home; you want the food to be part of what makes the occasion memorable. The same thing happens on holidays. Cranberry sauce, mashed potatoes, and yams are nothing special during the rest of the year, but on Thanksgiving they become delicious favorites because they are imbued with so much spirit and celebration.

We remember our holiday meals, of course, not only because of what we put on our plate but because of with whom we dine. Holidays are the few times when we surround ourselves with family and friends, give thanks for each other and the blessings we receive, and linger around the table. We take our time to eat, we lean back in our chairs, we laugh and enjoy the company of people we love. This environment transforms the way we eat (although sometimes we eat too much!) and calls our attention to an activity we usually take for granted.

Clearly we cannot make every meal such an occasion. But we can bring some of that awareness, love, and spirit into our daily lives. Whether you are eating a simple salad or a magnificent holiday meal, you can eat with the same awareness, the same presence of spirit and energy.

During the Wellness Rx week, make your meals an occasion for relaxing and focusing your attention away from problems and toward pleasures. Do not eat in front of the television. If you regularly eat in front of the television, turn it off and move to another room. If you read the newspaper while you eat, put it away and instead listen to some calm and soothing music. This has been shown to help people lose weight because it slows down the meal, making one less likely to overeat. Do not eat in the car on your way to work, or in between phone calls at the office.

Liven up your trips to the grocery store. If possible, find a natural-foods store that sells fresh produce. If you live in a rural area, visit a local farmer for farm-fresh fruits and vegetables. Ambitious readers may feel inclined to start their own garden of vegetables on a small plot of land in the backyard. Nothing could be more wonderful for you! Squashes, carrots, zucchinis, and watermelons are among the easiest foods to grow, and there is no end to the satisfaction of eating vegetables grown with your own hands. Most readers should be content to spend more time in the produce aisles, selecting fruits and vegetables with care, looking for color, shape, fragrance, and freshness.

Similarly, prepare your food with awareness. Pay attention to what you put into your mouth, even if you are just eating an apple. Stir your morning oatmeal with the same love that your mother or your grandmother felt when they did the same thing. Think about what you are eating; take time to really taste it. While you spend time in the kitchen, listen to some uplifting music, something you can sing along with. You will notice a difference in the food you make—it will taste more lively—and you will feel more satisfied, "soul-filled" rather than "full."

If it is still hard for you to imagine how it is that your attitude is an important ingredient in the foods you cook, I recommend you read the magnificent novel by Laura Esquivel *Like Water for Chocolate* or see the recent movie version. It is the story of a woman whose passionate and unhindered love flavors everything she prepares and affects the people who eat her food in profound ways!

The secret ingredient in any recipe, it seems, is that it be cooked with joy. Joy underlies all of the recipes presented for your convenience in the "Garden of Eating" portion of this book. At least for the Wellness Rx week, make an effort to fill your kitchen with joy as you cook. In doing so, you will feed your soul exactly what it is starving for, and in the process you will enhance your energy and strengthen your natural inner healer.

A Word About Vitamins

New information and discoveries about the benefits and limitations of vitamins, minerals, and antioxidants appear in the news nearly every week. It is virtually impossible to keep up with the broadening base of knowledge about dietary supplements. It is clear, however, that the traditional medical approach to vitamins has been inadequate. Every youthful medical student has heard this basic message from their biochemistry professor: "Patients don't need extra vitamins. They just need to have a balanced diet." The more cynical medical view is that patients who take vitamins are just enriching their urine and the vitamin companies.

New research suggests otherwise. I recommend that you take a multivitamin and mineral supplement each day. The fact is, the majority of people don't eat enough of the proper foods. Moreover, medications, lifestyle, habits, and emotional stress may drain you of essential nutrients even if you are eating the right foods. The recommended daily allowances (RDAs) were established decades ago and no longer reflect our changing needs.

How many vitamins should you take? Which kinds? The optimal formula lies somewhere in between the minimal levels recommended by traditional medical science and the megalevels suggested by "vitamin nuts" and industry spokespeople. This basic formula works for me and is the same formula I recommend to my patients of all ages: I purchase the least expensive generic equivalent to Centrum-Silver™, Theragran-M™, or GNC Daily Multivitamins and Minerals™ and instead of taking one tablet or capsule a day, I take two of them. I also take a baby aspirin each day for its protective effect against heart attack and stroke. If you are middle-aged or beyond, ask your doctor if there is any reason why you should not take a daily baby aspirin too.

If you have a particular illness or physical condition, ask your doctor if there are specific vitamin supplements that would be more appropriate for you to take, such as iron supplements for women in general and calcium supplements for menopausal women.

THE SUPER WELLNESS MEAL PLAN

To recap, the guidelines for eating during the week of the Wellness Rx are simply these:

Until Noon

- Eat as much fresh fruit and juice as you want.
- Eat whole-grain breads and cereals.
- Drink no more than two cups of caffeinated coffee and tea.
- If necessary, eat eggs only without the yolk.

Afternoon and Evening

- Substitute small amounts of chicken and fish for red meat.
- Limit red meat to no more than once this week, but preferably not at all.
- Reduce high-fat dairy foods such as cheese, butter, and ice cream. Choose non- or low-fat dairy products instead and drink no more than two 8-ounce glasses of nonfat milk.
- Eat primarily pasta, rice, baked potatoes, whole-grain breads, beans,

salads, and as many vegetables as you want
(raw, steamed, or lightly sautéed).
- Follow the recipes from the "Garden of Eating."
- Eat in a comfortable, relaxed environment; turn off the television, fold away the paper, and concentrate on *enjoying* your food.
- Make love your secret ingredient.
- Cook and eat with **JOY!**

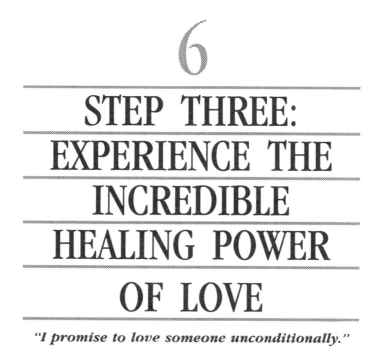

6

STEP THREE: EXPERIENCE THE INCREDIBLE HEALING POWER OF LOVE

"I promise to love someone unconditionally."

Mother Teresa, praised by millions of people around the world, has written that "we have all been created for the sole purpose to love and be loved." The success of the Wellness Rx is rooted in part in the recognition that your sole purpose, and your *soul* purpose, is love. Beneath all illness lies a longing for love, an ache for that powerful force that dwells in our hearts and joins us to the heart of heaven. Love is what your soul craves. Nothing influences your well-being and health more profoundly than love—not only the love that you receive but especially the love that you give away freely, without condition.

There is no shield that provides more powerful protection from illness and disease than love. When we are loving and feel loved, we experience a wholeness in our lives that heals the feelings of isolation and separation that we all perceive from time to time. In those moments of wholeness, the body's energy is perfectly balanced, and there is no *disease*. That presence of wholeness can be achieved only by you. Wholeness cannot be prescribed by your physician, and it does not come from external intervention. Wholeness is born of the soul and is nurtured by love. Love is the Healing Force of your inner physician, that magnificent system of energy that is far more powerful than all of scientific medicine.

You may say, "I have enough love; what I need now is to heal." Or, you may think, "How can I love someone else unconditionally when right now I need to concentrate all of my love on myself to get better?" You may even be thinking silently to yourself, "I am ill or tired because I am not loved enough. How can I give away more love than I am receiving?" The answers are not simple, but they are close. Indeed, the answers lie within each and every one of us, hidden in our souls.

The soul craves love. You may long for another person's love—a lover or spouse, a parent, a child—but the soul longs only for your love, which it feels when you are loving toward others. How often we ask for love to come into our lives and free us from boredom, misery, or loneliness. But how often do we ask, Who is in need of my love right now? When you offer your love unconditionally to someone else, your soul is drenched in joy and the Healing Force sings. That song of the soul reverberates through every single cell of your body and brings balance, harmony, and the reverence for life that are essential to your wellness.

HOW LOVE HEALS TODAY'S MOST COMMON AILMENTS

Health, as I have described it, is essentially a spiritual journey. Our lives throughout this journey are spent in fluctuation along a continuum somewhere between wholeness and isolation. When we feel a sense of wholeness, we are strong spiritually, and that strength enhances the inherent healing processes that occur in every living person. The experience of isolation has precisely the opposite effect. Social isolation is felt deep within the soul. Without a sense of connectedness to other lives and a greater purpose, reverence for life diminishes and the Healing Force grows dim. This spiritual longing is the ground on which the seeds of physical illness sprout. Before we can heal physical ailments, we need to address the emotional and spiritual aches that isolation entails. This is true whether you have problems of asthma, arthritis, alcoholism, weight disorders, back pain, migraine, insomnia, colitis, depression, chronic fatigue or even cancer. In every instance, the wholeness and feeling of connectedness that offering your unconditional love generates will enhance your ability to heal. Even if **full** recovery is not immediately likely, as in the case of AIDS, your potential to overcome the pain and suffering that accompany illness is immeasurably increased when your soul responds to the act of offering your love unconditionally.

So for the week of the Wellness Rx, agree to love someone you know unconditionally. The person to whom you choose to give your unconditional love can be anyone: a parent, spouse, child, relative, friend, or neighbor—even a family pet. What matters most is not the person you choose to unconditionally love but the content of this love. *Unconditionally* means without conditions. There are no boundaries of unconditional love, no disappointments, no disputes.

This is the love that Albert Schweitzer had in mind when he wrote, "Love cannot be put under a system of rules and regulations. It issues absolute commands." To love someone unconditionally is to love them entirely for who they are, faults and all. Loving unconditionally means that no matter what someone said or did that made you angry or upset, you recognize that all of those feelings cannot compare with the feeling of love you have for that person. Whether you choose your child, spouse, parent, sibling, or coworker, for one week, let nothing that they do, no matter how infuriating or insensitive, change the fact that you are practicing loving them unconditionally. And the response of love in any situation overpowers all other forms of response, especially anger.

CASE HISTORY—FRANK'S FIGHT FOR LOVE

Frank is a fifty-four-year-old patient who came to me because he was suffering with blinding migraine headaches at least two or three times a week, and they were unresponsive to at least a dozen medicines that he had been on. Frank worked on an assembly line at a factory and feared losing his job because of absenteeism due to the headaches. He was anxious to begin the Wellness Rx but skeptical that he would succeed at the promise of loving someone unconditionally. There were so many people, according to his account, who drove him "nuts" daily that choosing any single person to love unconditionally seemed impossible. "None of them are going to make this very easy," he said. Although I sympathized with his efforts to select the person in his life who might be easiest to love unconditionally, I had to explain to him that he was missing the point. Loving someone unconditionally means looking beyond all of those annoying words, habits, or attitudes and seeing, essentially, just another soul.

In his wife, his daughter, and his mother, Frank saw just a messy mixture of irritating behaviors. "My wife bugs me about the old car I'm fixing up in the driveway. She's going crazy about the oil stains on the cement." "Just the way my daughter looks at me bothers me, like she's trying to figure out how to defy me." "Every time my brother comes around he's flaunting some new merchandise or something just to remind me he makes more money than me." And so on, and so on. Trying to get Frank to look beyond these irritations to see his family members as souls was not going to be easy. There were so many layers upon layers of attitudes, emotions, beliefs, hurts, angers, frustrations, and disappointments piled up around them that in his eyes their shrouded souls seemed like tiny specks of light in the distance of a dark and dusty tunnel.

But Frank was a religious man. He was a member of the Baptist church and basically felt in his heart that every person was made in the image of God. Could Frank see this reflection of God within his individual family members? "I guess I'd have to say I haven't thought of them in that way for a real long time."

For Frank, unconditionally loving someone meant learning to see in that person again a reflection of a Higher Power. He felt strongly that if this were going to be a promise he could keep, to love someone unconditionally for one week, he had to start where there was the greatest possibility of success. He chose his daughter Kay, a fifteen-year-old who was preoccupied with cars, late nights, and the movies. Frank believed that anytime he asked Kay for some help around the house or yard, feeding the animals or taking out the trash, she only gave in with a grudge. "She thinks it's a big deal if I even ask her to clean up her room." On top of that, Frank felt Kay did everything she was asked to do only halfway, and in the manner most exactly the opposite of how her father would do it, just to anger him. "She's always doing things just to make some sort of point, like she knows better than me."

For the first Wellness Rx week, Frank made a personal promise to love his daughter unconditionally. If Kay hesitated or complained when Frank asked her to clean up the backyard, Frank promised not to respond with anger or sarcasm. No matter how frustrating Kay's behavior was, Frank promised to try to convey the fact that he still loved her unconditionally. After one week, Frank returned to my office to describe his week. I asked him about his diet and exercise, but he skipped right to his promise of unconditional love. "It feels good, you know? I'm not sure why, but it is so much easier now than it was to get along with Kay." "Are you being more gentle with her?" I asked. "Oh yes," he responded. "Well, and she is more gentle with me." I asked Frank why he thought his daughter's behavior might have changed so much in one week. "She is seeing that the things she does just have no effect on me. You know, before I would see her do something, just piddling little stuff that didn't amount to anything and I would ask her 'Why do you do it that way?' I don't even notice that now." "Do you feel more love for her?" I asked. "Oh yes," he replied. "Just taking my mind off how angry she makes me strengthened that love. Everytime I thought of getting angry, I said to myself, 'See the reflection of God in her.' How can I be angry at that?"

Because Frank's migraines were so frequent and severe, we extended the Wellness Rx to two weeks. During that second week, Frank knew he had to promise to love his wife unconditionally, since the problems they were having communicating seemed to be a major contribution to his headaches. Frank openly admitted that he was raised to think of women, as he put it, as "sort of inferior." After promising to love his wife unconditionally for a week, which meant in this case seeing her as his equal, Frank agreed that this promise was crucial to overcoming his headaches.

When he returned a week later, he looked years younger, and the dark rings around his eyes were gone. "I'm following all my promises, but especially I'm seeing more God in my wife," he told me. "She is kind of like the flowers after they bloom. You know, until this week, I was seeing her before they got into full bloom." I asked how the communication between them was going since he had started loving her unconditionally. "Until this week, it seemed like we really had to force ourselves to find something to say, like we have said everything in the last twenty years that there was to say. Mostly we just snapped at each other or I was complaining about her or she was going on about me. But this week has been so smooth, and we actually seem to be enjoying each other's company." Frank cracked the first smile I had seen since he walked in my office two weeks earlier.

Frank's relationship with his family, especially his views about women, still required a lot of mending. I am happy to report, however, that one year after the Wellness Rx, the frequency of Frank's migraine attacks has lessened from two or three times every week to just once or twice a year—and that he dearly loves his wife and daughter again.

Even those who seem the most disagreeable to you deserve your unconditional love. A coworker who annoys you, a relative, or the stubborn checkout clerk at the grocery store—each is worthy of your unconditional love. "All God's angels," wrote James Russell Lowell, "come to us disguised." The Bible says nearly the same thing: "Be not forgetful to entertain strangers, for thereby some have entertained angels unawares." Or, as Frank discovered, many people are flowers that would bloom, if only they were illumined by the sunlight of our love.

Unconditional love should be offered selflessly. Remember, there are no conditions to this kind of love. To be truly unconditional, this love is offered without expectations of anything in return. If you choose to love someone unconditionally because you want their unconditional love in return, you are already placing a condition on the love you give. Unconditional love means expecting *nothing* in return.

Loving selflessly, however, does not mean that you gain nothing and give everything. Indeed, there are very potent health benefits to loving unconditionally, as I will explain in a moment. The key, however, is that you are not offering your unconditional love for any kind of personal gain. Offer love only out of love. Love that is offered out of personal gain is fine, but it is not unconditional. Unconditionally love your mother, your daughter, your husband, or whomever, because you want to love them unconditionally, not because you expect to gain from doing so. Love for love's sake.

THE LOVE-HEALTH CONNECTION

Love that is given in this manner, selflessly, purely out of love, and without condition, automatically enhances your body's natural-healing resources. Loving someone unconditionally nurtures your soul and brings balance to your feelings and emotions. Loving someone truly unconditionally enhances your reverence for life, your self-worth, and your sense of purpose. These attributes are much more than "health benefits." Reverence for life, self-worth, and purpose are the cornerstones of a life of wholeness and balance, forever. When you live your life in this balance, with this wholeness, illness cannot harm you.

But good health is only one of the effects of living soulfully, with soul purpose. That soul purpose expands far beyond establishing health and wellness. Good health is a point along the journey, but it is not the final destination. The journey is soulward, into the source from which we were born, soulful. Unconditional love is one of the most direct paths soulward. Love determines the success of our effort to return to the soul. As Henry Thoreau knew so well, "There must be the generating force of love behind every effort destined to be successful." Unconditional love opens up a window to the soul, whose light, like a compass, draws us inward, soulward, where we belong.

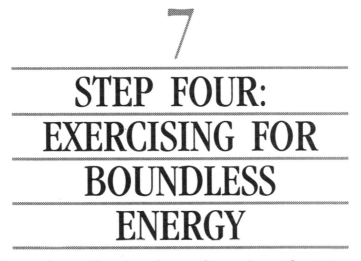

7

STEP FOUR:
EXERCISING FOR
BOUNDLESS
ENERGY

"I promise to do some form of exercise at least twenty minutes a day this week."

When was the last time you felt playful? When was the last time you swam in the ocean or sledded down a snowy hill? When was the last time you "cut a rug" dancing to a fast rhythm? Are you so busy that you think there is no time for fun in your life? If you answered yes to this last question or could not remember enough to answer the previous questions, then surely you are in need of the Wellness Rx. You need it because exercise is the absolute linchpin of health and energy, and also because the ability to be playful is essential to cultivating a deep reverence for life.

Exercise is the single most important step that you can take toward achieving the balance of energy that defines your personal wellness. We commonly think of exercise as something that "burns energy," because we think of exercise in terms of burning calories, which are energy. But exercise not only burns up energy; more important, it produces new and greater amounts of energy. And by drawing energy into the body, exercise helps establish the balance required for healing and wellness.

Now I am not necessarily referring to the kind of intense workout regimen that you approach with the same seriousness associated with work. Indeed, too much exercise, or exercise of such intensity as to provoke exhaustion, actually depletes your energy supply, in which case the body turns to other sources for its much-needed energy, breaking down its own tissues and thereby stressing your balance of energy.

The kind of "workout" the Wellness Rx entails is one that takes the work *out* of playing and having fun. The best kind of exercise for your health is any physical activity that makes you breathe a little bit faster, that makes you laugh and smile, and that is filled with a sense of play. Nothing ignites the Healing Force more immediately, and my patients unanimously agree that this kind of exercise is the turning point in their journey to wellness. Paradoxically, because we generally associate exercise with rigorous work, it is also almost always the first promise that most people will avoid fulfilling.

Exercising well means tossing out the unrealistic regimens, far-fetched goals, and negative thought patterns about exercise that prime you for a disappointing experience with exercise. My patients are surprised at how flexible the exercise component of this program is. One patient, a dairy farmer, was concerned about meeting this requirement and confided in me that he had not exercised since gym class in high school.

"Doctor, the only exercise I get is chasing the cows around."
"How long does it take you to do that?" I asked.
"A good twenty minutes, depending on how stubborn they're feeling."
"And does that make you work up a sweat?"
"Heck yes! Have you ever tried chasing twenty-five cows out into the field?"
"Fine," I said. "All that matters is that whatever physical activity you do, it elevates your heart rate, quickens your breath, and works up a little sweat."

Chasing cows for twenty minutes provides the same physiological and mental benefits that jogging a mile around a track does. Exercising no longer has to entail an expensive health club membership or a special wardrobe. The exercise promoted in the Wellness Rx asks you to do nothing more than work a moderate amount of exercise into your daily routine.

All of the attention the media has given to high-tech, high-speed workouts has raised the American consciousness about the importance of exercise. But for many, the "just-do-it" campaigns that feature high-impact, heavy-intensity exercises (always, of course, done by models and athletes fitting the current image of what is beautiful and "healthy," an image achievable by very few of us) may have been a discouraging message that exercise is for the already fit and hard-bodied. Rock climbing, step aerobics, and mountain biking are great. But they are not for everyone. And there are just as many easier ways to get the same benefits of exercise.

New guidelines from the American College of Sports Medicine, the Centers for Disease Control and Prevention, and the Council on Physical Fitness and Sports advocate small doses of exercise accumulated over the day, claiming that this approach is just as beneficial as one sustained workout. Five trips up several flights of stairs during the day, walking to and from your car parked a few blocks away from work or shopping, raking leaves, or gardening can provide enough physical exertion to stimulate physiological changes and promote wellness.

WHY EXERCISE STRENGTHENS YOUR IMMUNE SYSTEM

New studies show that even the smallest increase in physical activity, the difference between taking the elevator or climbing five flights of stairs, lowers your risks of developing heart disease, hypertension, diabetes, osteoporosis, obesity, breast cancer, and colon cancer. Small doses of exercise are especially important to neutralizing the destructive thought patterns of depression, anxiety, stress, worry, panic, and anger that contribute so significantly to our physiological illnesses.

Why does exercise contribute so significantly to wellness and balance? Even moderate movement bolsters the immune system's defenses against illness. Exercise triggers the increased production of your body's natural healing agents, the natural killer cells and serum immunoglobulins, substances that ward off potential illness. Research actually suggests that too much exercise, or exercise pushed to the point of stress, increases another substance known to depress the ability of immune cells to do their job. The key to a successful exercise program that will deliver the health benefits and mental clarity integral to the Wellness Rx is *moderation*.

The word from Washington early this year was that Americans are facing an "epidemic of physical inactivity." According to the government, half of the adult population prefers snoozing to stretching, kicking back to kicking it up. The Centers for Disease Control and Prevention estimate that nearly 60 percent of Americans eighteen and older are sedentary— "couch potatoes." That means that 60 percent of us are placing ourselves at greater risk for heart disease, hypertension, osteoporosis, diabetes, and cancer. Indeed, an estimated 250,000 Americans die yearly because of illnesses related to inactivity.

The couch potato phenomenon is understandable, given a decade of hard-body hype that very few of us actually could, or should, aspire to. Many of us face self-defeat before we even lace up our new Reeboks™. Between what work demands and what our children need, where is that extra hour for an aerobics class to be found? Not to mention the extra money required to join an expensive health club.

Exercising well means shattering the myth that you need a gym membership and the latest gear to be fit. It also means that you no longer need to search for an extra hour in the day to get your exercise. Exercising well is as simple as working twenty or more minutes of moderate activity into your day. There are no restrictions on what kinds of activity you do, just that you do it for an accumulated total of twenty minutes and that it gets you a little bit huffy and puffy.

Now all of this is not to say throw away your mountain bikes, get rid of your hiking boots, and put away the tennis rackets. On the contrary, if you are already a physically active person, continue the exercise routine you are presently doing. The point here is not to say that running is bad; rather, the message is that walking is *just as good* in terms of stimulating the immune system and preventing disease.

NINE EASY WAYS TO RECHARGE YOUR BATTERIES

You might be surprised at what falls into the category of exercise given these new guidelines endorsed by top exercise physiologists and specialists. The possibilities for fulfilling this promise of the Wellness Rx are endless. Here are several ways of working exercise into your everyday life without going out of your way.

- Forget the elevator; take the stairs instead.
- Park a few blocks away from work or shopping and walk the remaining distance at a quick pace.
- Take a fifteen-minute walk during lunch (just bring a pair of walking shoes to change into).
- Play tag outdoors with your child or a neighbor's child. Consult a child for more ideas!

- Take your child to a nearby playground and run around playing on the different gym equipment. (Pushing even a lightweight child on a swing is a great way to strengthen your arms, shoulders, and chest.)
- Work in the garden, pulling weeds or raking leaves. (To protect your back, be sure to bend at the knees rather than at your waist.)
- Walk your dog.
- Go dancing (no high heels!).
- Dribble a basketball or kick around a soccerball.

Do one of these activities, or some combination of them. You do not need to do a full twenty minutes all at once, just as long as the small periods of activity add up to around twenty minutes by the end of the day.

CASE HISTORY—SUZANNE'S STORY

Suzanne, a thirty-three-year-old executive at an advertising agency, was a prime candidate for the Wellness Rx. Her father was a diabetic and her mother had arthritis. Suzanne had a mild case of chronic irritable bowel syndrome. Milk exacerbated her symptoms (alternating periods of constipation, diarrhea, gassiness, and abdominal pain), and alcohol made them intolerable. Ice cream and wine were her only weaknesses. Suzanne was slightly over her optimal weight and was concerned that starting birth control pills would encourage further weight gain. She was generally motivated, enthusiastic, and seemed naturally cheerful. She was already beginning to make the changes prescribed in the Wellness Rx program when she walked into my office. Working out the details with her was simple, until we got to the part about exercise.

On her patient questionnaire Suzanne indicated that currently she was not doing any kind of exercise. I told her that moderate exercise would be key to overcoming her condition.

"Forget it, Doctor. There is no way I can promise to exercise. It's not that I wouldn't like to exercise; it's just that twenty minutes of doing nothing is a real luxury right now in my busy schedule. I can't possibly afford the time."

Suzanne then went on to describe her tight schedule. "I work in the city, where driving is crazy and parking is so scarce that I take the commuter train into work. But the closest stop to my office is three blocks away, so I'm running behind before I even reach the building."

I interrupted her story right there. "Do you take the commuter train home as well?"

"Yes, and unless I want to be stuck in the city until dark, I have to get there by five, which is really pushing it. I bring running shoes just so I can move faster."

"So you walk three blocks twice a day?"

"I wouldn't call it walking; it's more like running because I'm always rushing to get here or there. It takes me exactly ten point five minutes each way—a minute too slow and I miss the train."

So it seemed that Suzanne was already getting the dose of exercise she needed. When I pointed this out she was amazed. I suggested that all that she had to do now was to get a good pair of walking shoes, give herself some credit for taking morning and evening exercise walks, make a concerted effort to clear her mind during that walking time rather than trying to plan her busy work schedule, and take the stairs instead of the elevator at work. "Walk with awareness," I advised her. "Put your total effort into it, and see if you don't notice any changes."

Suzanne returned a week later, at the end of her Wellness Rx, even more bright and lively than just six days earlier. She was also three pounds lighter and her symptoms were dramatically reduced, which was probably related to the fact that she was drinking more water to compensate for what she lost during her exercising. "Just putting my mind into my walks made them more invigorating. I love my new walking shoes so much I wear them all day when I'm behind the desk. I stopped using the elevator at work. I have so much more energy throughout the rest of the day now, and I look forward to my walk at the end of the day."

With the Wellness Rx, you can turn any activity you already do regularly into moderate exercise and still get all of the health benefits you need from exercise.

THE ELEVEN AMAZING BENEFITS OF WALKING

Walking is the most versatile form of exercise there is. The possibilities for making fun out of walking are limitless. So are the benefits. Besides stimulating your immune system and increasing your energy, walking regularly promotes the following results:

- Enhances your stamina and aerobic capacity

- Reduces fat in your bloodstream
- Increases your muscle flexibility
- Strengthens your heart
- Keeps your knee and hip joints supple
- Helps prevent brittle bones
- Lowers blood pressure
- Encourages weight loss
- Enhances your sexuality
- Relieves lower-back tension
- Works out stress

The benefits of exercise simply cannot be overstated, particularly concerning weight loss. A study reported by scientists at Tufts University involved a group of men and women in their sixties divided into two groups: subjects who exercised and subjects who went on a specific diet. Each person in the exercise group was required to burn up to 360 calories a day on a stationary bike while those in the diet group were required to eat 360 less calories a day than they were used to eating. According to basic math, both groups should have lost the same amount of weight during the study. The researchers were stunned to find instead that people who did exercise without dieting lost 50 percent more weight than those who dieted without exercising. The exercisers lost more pure fatty tissue than dieters: 400 percent more! Numerous studies concur that exercise is the major key to weight loss and a trim, lean physique. Less exercise means more fat. More exercise means less flab.

There are many ways to make a walk enjoyable. My patients agree that some of their most creative moments come when they are walking. Walking not only gets the muscles flexing and the blood surging, it gets ideas flowing. Here are just three suggestions that my patients have enjoyed:

1. Walk in a beautiful place nearby: a park, a beach, a forest, or just a quiet street where there is not much traffic. Walk with an awareness of your surroundings. Notice trees and the color of leaves, notice wildflowers growing out of the cracks in the sidewalk beneath your feet, observe the scenery around you. Walk briskly, but not in such a rush that you overlook these things. As you walk, think to yourself, "I am surrounded by Nature's healing presence."

2. As you walk, listen to uplifting or motivating music on a portable cassette player. Select music that literally *moves* you, whether it is reggae, classical, inspirational, baroque, country, or Gregorian chants. My patients have found that listening to the radio is not as good because the commercials slow them down and are distracting. Let the rhythm of the music carry you along. Walk with good posture, arms swinging, as if you were conducting the orchestra, band, or choir you are listening to. Walk with intention, purpose, will. Feel the orchestra of your body—your arms, legs, head, back, stomach, feet—playing and moving totally in harmony as blood and energy flow to each muscle in your body.

3. Walk with someone you care for or love!

YOGA—NATURE'S WAY TO NEW FLEXIBILITY AND STRENGTH

To increase energy and to balance energy, no form of exercise is more effective than hatha yoga. For the week of the Wellness Rx, you are required to practice yoga on at least two occasions. You can practice yoga in addition to or instead of the more vigorous form of exercise you choose. Don't worry about flexibility, because the recommended postures are very easy to do. I chose them with myself in mind, and I am very, very unflexible—but still working on it.

Hatha yoga is the physical branch of the scientific system of yoga. It is based on a series of physical postures, or asanas, literally thousands of positions developed in ancient India around the eleventh century. During the last three decades, yoga practices have been incorporated into a Western approach to stretching and exercise. Today, yoga is taught in health clubs, community centers, and universities as a form of "stress management" and is practiced in tens of thousands of homes across the country. No longer stigmatized as an exercise for "hippies" or "wimps," yoga has attained widespread popularity particularly among corporate executives, pregnant women, professional athletes, nationally renowned physicians, and college students.

Why the growing interest in yoga? People across the country are recognizing the health benefits of yoga. Not only does it reduce stress, but regular practice of even a few yoga positions cultivates muscular strength, flexibility in the spine and muscles, improved circulation, expanded lung capacity, healthy digestion, and prevents the joints and bones from becoming stiff and brittle. Yoga postures do much more than stretch and strengthen muscles. Many positions work far beneath the layers of skin and muscle, stimulating internal organs such as the stomach and regions of the digestive tract. Other positions, such as the simple inverted postures (introduced below), place a gentle, subtle pressure on the thyroid gland, which helps to stimulate metabolism and energy. Indeed, yoga works the entire body, and millions of people are experiencing its physiological benefits.

There is another, perhaps more significant reason why Americans are turning to yoga. People are trying out yoga not only because they are more exercise aware, or more health conscious in general, but because they are responding to their soul's inner call. If running is a "workout," then yoga might be thought of as a "work within." Yoga soothes and expands the soul. And the most amazing thing about yoga is that it does this even if that is not particularly your goal. Indeed, most people begin practicing yoga to improve their flexibility or muscle tone, but after only a few weeks, they cannot ignore the deeper inner awareness that accompanies the physical postures.

THE HEALING POWERS OF YOGA

After a month of practicing yoga to help alleviate chronic back pain, Mary, a fifty-seven-year-old patient, wrote me a wonderful letter:

> These stretching and flexing exercises are miraculous! The ache in my lower back is nearly gone, after years of causing me such pain I could hardly bend. But that's not the only miracle. I don't know what it is about the exercises, but since I started doing them, I feel an inner calm, like a spiritual presence that I've never had before. It's like my soul just opened up.

Now, Mary is hardly a "New-Age" person and she is a devout member of the same Catholic church she grew up in. I never told her to expect the yoga postures to affect her at a spiritual level, because I knew that might hinder her willingness to practice these exercises for her back. But like most of my patients who practice even small amounts of yoga, she could not help but feel how the exercises reached deep within her and opened up her soul as they stretched out her back. Most people start doing yoga for physical benefits and stress management. They are pleasantly surprised when they discover changes in their emotional and spiritual outlook.

Yoga is more than a physical workout. Yoga works the whole body, mind, and soul. It engages your muscles, your thoughts, your feelings, and your attitudes. Yoga enhances your health because it works at all these levels. At the same time that it releases tension and tightness in the muscles, it releases harmful emotions and painful feelings that can lead to illness. Indeed, because the Wellness Rx is designed to alleviate the underlying *causes* of illness, and not just its physical *symptoms*, yoga makes perfect sense as a strategy for wellness. Yoga eases back pain not just by stretching the muscles and strengthening the spine but by subtly releasing the underlying soul ache that defines the physical pain (this is addressed in more detail in Chapter Fifteen, on overcoming backache). Back pain, migraine, arthritis, colitis, chronic fatigue, and hypertension will be only temporarily relieved until those deeper aches are tended to.

Yoga comes from the Sanskrit word *yogah*, which means "union" or "to unite." *Hatha* means "balance." Every yoga posture was created to reflect and inspire these underlying principles of union and balance. The reason why yoga affects us both physically and spiritually is that the postures come from and help create union between these dimensions. Unlike the exercise trends in the United States, which are driven by physical benefits, yoga speaks to the entire body, mind, and soul, because in India, where yoga originates, there is no separation between the physical and the mental. In fact, this split makes no sense within the cultural framework from which yoga emerges.

The Wellness Rx is a seven-day "timeout" developed to re-create and strengthen the balance of energy in your body. Yoga is an excellent activity because it fosters that balance. Once you have established the inner balance of energy, you become like a sturdy sailboat, and no winds of stress or illness can shake you off course. But when that balance withers, your sails become shaky, and the slightest stress can throw you entirely off balance, causing you to become ill.

Yoga is perfect for you if the idea of sweaty, huffing and puffing exercise does not appeal to you. It is also an ideal fitness activity for those who live in cold, rainy, or snowy climates where going outdoors for a walk or gardening may not be practical.

Asthma Relief

Stewart, a forty-seven-year-old patient, suffered greatly from asthma since he was a child. His wheezing and shortness of breath were much worse in the spring pollen season and always bad when he was under work deadlines—which happened to be most of the time. A vast array of medications never proved to be of much relief.

Stewart had great difficulty keeping his exercise promise until he tried yoga. Prior to that, he just found it too hard to sustain even fifteen minutes of a more traditional fitness regimen of weights and the stationary bicycle. But then this busy Hollywood studio executive followed a friend to a yoga class. Now he does yoga in his home five days a week, an hour each day. Not bad for a person who could not make it through even fifteen minutes of more intense exercise.

I saw Stewart for a follow-up visit three months after he first came to my office. His lungs sounded remarkably clear, not like the lungs of a person with severe asthma. Stewart explained his new progress.

"I thought I had to lift massive weights to build strength. I had no idea how much yoga builds strength and endurance." But Stewart found much more to yoga than physical strength.

"I like the changes in my body since I've been doing yoga, but more exciting to me are the changes in my mental attitude and spiritual outlook. Everyone around me has noticed how calm I've become, which is tough to say in this town."

An important aspect of yoga is that it helps cultivate awareness or mindfulness in your life. In the same way that you are asked to eat with an awareness of energy during the Wellness Rx, practicing yoga transforms your awareness into energy of the body. Yoga requires concentration. You may be able to read a magazine while you peddle away at a stationary bike, but you will not be able to hold a yoga position and read or listen to your Walkman™ at the same time. Yoga may appear to be a passive activity that does not require much effort. You may even have seen someone doing a yoga posture on television and thought how boring that looks just sitting there. Exactly the opposite is true, because yoga requires not only physical coordination but mental focus. This is one reason why Stewart liked yoga so much. "When I do yoga, it is impossible for me to think of anything else but what I am doing at that moment. At every other moment of the day my mind is jumping from here to there. Yoga brings my mind into the present."

HOW YOGA CAN DISSOLVE NEGATIVE FEELINGS

When your mind is in the present, in the "here and now," stressful events do not have to rattle and shake you up. Emotional responses to stress are triggered not by what is happening right now, this instant, but what has already happened or what we fear may happen in the future. Remorse, regret, guilt, anticipation, anxiety, suspense, expectation—these feelings pull us into the past or plunge us into the future. None of these things are tied to the present. Most people actually spend very little time in the present moment. How often does your mind drift into your memory or ahead in time as you read this very page?

Our minds are on overload, constantly shuttling back and forth at chaotic speeds and with seemingly no coherence between what has been and what will be. Have you ever noticed what you think about as you are lying in bed ready to fall asleep? "I need to get gas before work in the morning . . . that meeting was so bad . . . what will I wear tomorrow? . . . I should have worn the blue suit yesterday . . . my mother would have hated that suit . . . I should call my mom tomorrow . . . when is her birthday? . . . What will I get her this year? . . . It can't be late again this year . . . I hope the check comes in the mail tomorrow . . . what is my current balance? . . . that exercise bike was too expensive; I should never have bought it . . . I'd like to buy that new car . . . I can't forget to stop for gas before work tomorrow . . . did I set the alarm?"

The other day I saw a bumper sticker that captured what I am getting at here: "It's five o'clock. Do you know where your mind is?"

When you do yoga, you know where your mind is because it is right in the posture, in the muscle you are stretching, following your breath. In those moments when your mind is not dragging in the past or running ahead of you into the future, the harmful emotions, feelings, beliefs, attitudes, memories, and desires that contribute to illness are neutralized. When those illness-inviting thoughts are distilled, your mind becomes a garden where wellness-inspiring thoughts of joy, connectedness, balance, and wholeness are cultivated.

The following yoga exercises will help you fulfill the exercise component of the Wellness Rx. They are geared toward the beginner, but those with greater flexibility and strength should not dismiss them as being too "easy." While there are some yoga postures that are "advanced," in general, the difference between a beginning level and an advanced level of yoga has less to do with specific postures and more to do with how long you can hold the posture and how deeply you are able to concentrate while doing it. Therefore, the postures here are suitable for people with no experience of yoga as well as for those who have practiced yoga previously. The difference is in how long you remain in a single position and how focused your mind becomes.

CREATING AN OASIS OF CALMNESS

Do yoga in a quiet setting. If you have children, do your postures before they wake in the morning or while they are at school. (Once you learn the poses yourself, you can teach them to your children—yoga is a great activity on which to focus all of that childhood energy!) If you work and do not have time during the morning, you may find that doing even one or two yoga positions before you go to bed will help you fall asleep more quickly and sleep more relaxed. Whenever you do yoga postures, wear loose-fitting clothing in which you can move and stretch comfortably. Listen to relaxing music if you wish, or open a window so you can feel the fresh air as you breath. Most important, listen to your body. Never push a stretch to the point of pain. And if you are currently under the care of your physician for any physical injury, consult him or her before beginning these exercises. Remember to do the yoga exercises at least two times during your week to wellness.

YOUR PERFECT YOGA ROUTINE—ELEVEN STEPS TOWARD REJUVENATION

Step 1: Sitting Pose

Sit comfortably on the floor with your legs crossed. Close your eyes and be aware of your posture. Sit up tall, lifting up through the spine. Relax your shoulders and draw your awareness into the present moment by focusing on your breath. Don't control your breathing; just be aware of it.

Step 2: Full Breath

Sitting comfortably and with good posture, eyes still closed, take a long, deep breath. As you inhale, relax your stomach muscles, then contract them as you exhale slowly. (This may be the opposite of how you regularly breathe. Many women, in particular, programmed to think a perfectly flat stomach is ideal, suck in their stomachs when they inhale. Breathing this way limits the oxygen capacity of the lower lungs.) Place your hand on your belly to feel the movement. The belly rises as you inhale, falls as you exhale. If it helps, imagine between your rib cage a balloon that fills with air as you inhale, expanding the chest and ribs, and releases air as you exhale. *Do the full breath five times slowly, counting to 3 on the inhale and 3 on the exhale.* (As your lung capacity increases, build up to five- and then seven-second inhalations and exhalations.)

Step 3: Gentle Neck Rotation

Still sitting with a long spine, shrug your shoulders up close to your ears. Gently and slowly roll your head to the left, then slowly around to the front, tucking the chin to chest, then slowly to the right, and finally back to center. *Do this three times in one direction, and then do three rotations in the reverse direction, slowly.*

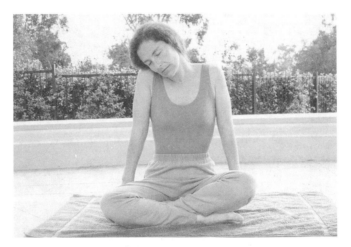

Gentle Neck Rotation 1

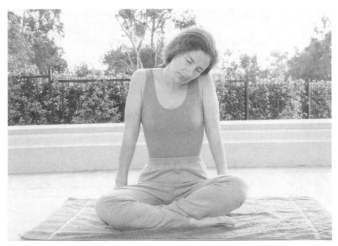

Gentle Neck Rotation 2

Step 4: Shoulder Shrugs

In the same sitting position, inhale deeply and shrug your shoulders up by your ears, squeezing them together. Hold for a count of three, then let them fall loosely as you exhale. Imagine as you do this that you are squeezing out the tension in your upper back and shoulders. *Do this three times.*

Step 5: The Cat Pose

This gentle posture stretches your back, strengthens your arms, and relaxes your upper back and neck. First, place your weight on your hands and knees, with your hands beneath your shoulders and your knees directly beneath your hips. Take a deep breath, and as you exhale, curl your back toward the ceiling, just like a cat stretching. As you curl your back, tuck your chin closely to your chest. *Hold for five seconds, breathing deeply.* Next, slowly flatten out your back and raise your chin to look straight ahead, and as you inhale, arch your spine gently, making a small dip in the middle back. Keep your elbows straight and your head relaxed. *Alternate between the curled and arched positions three times slowly.*

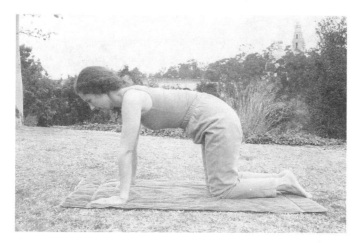

Cat Pose 1

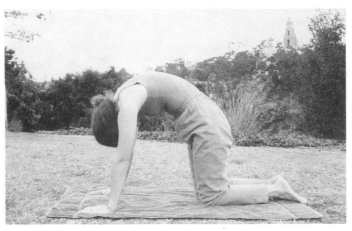

Cat Pose 2

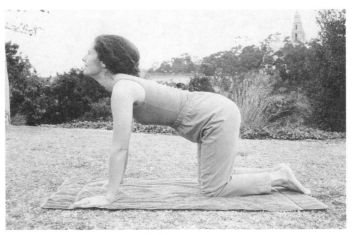

Cat Pose 3

Step 6: The Cobra

Stretch out on the floor, lying on your belly. Let your legs relax against the floor, your arms lying comfortably by your side. Inhale deeply and lift your chin off the ground, tilting your head slightly (do not overextend your neck). Bend your elbows and bring your hands to rest just beneath your shoulders. Take another deep breath and gently press the palms of your hands against the floor and lift your upper body off the floor. Exhale, and be sure you are not straining your neck. Squeeze your stomach and buttocks muscles to protect your lower back. You should feel a stretch in the lower and middle back. *Hold this posture for three full breaths.* Relax your upper body back to the floor and loosen your stomach and buttocks muscles. Rest your head on one cheek and take a few more breaths here, letting your back relax.

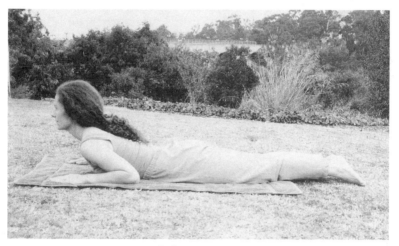

Cobra Pose 1

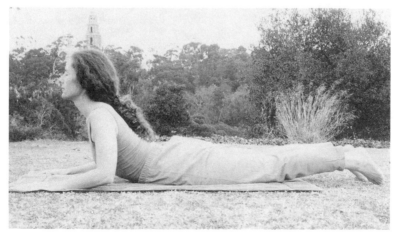

Cobra Pose 2

Step 7: The Rag Doll

Stand tall and with correct posture: feet a few inches apart with your weight evenly distributed across both, shoulders relaxed, knees soft. Inhale, then exhale, tucking your chin to your chest and slowly begin to curl your body forward, loosely, like a rag doll. Curl the upper body down slowly, until you are bending softly at the waist, your upper body hanging loosely over your legs. You should be staring at your knees. Let your arms sway as your upper body relaxes, limp and free of tension. (Do not lock your knees.) Take three deep breaths here. With bent knees, slowly begin to come back up, one vertebrae at a time, keeping your chin tucked until you are standing straight up. Breathe deeply in the standing position, with your eyes closed, and feel how relaxed your body is.

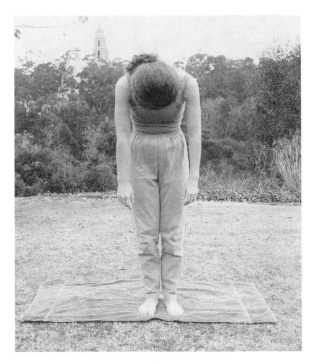

Rag Doll Pose 1

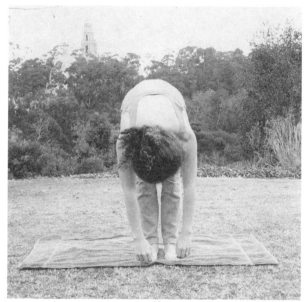

Rag Doll Pose 2

Step 8: The Half Moon

This pose strengthens your lower back, abdominals, and obliques (the muscles along your sides) and increases flexibility in the spine. Standing tall, inhale and raise your arms out to the side and up above your head, placing your palms together in a "prayer" position. Check your posture; make sure your pelvis is tucked and your knees are not locked. Now, inhale and stretch up onto your toes, lengthening your whole body. As you lower back down onto the flats of your feet, slowly bend sideways to the left, letting your hips go to the right as you stretch your arms over your head to the left. Keep your lower back and stomach muscles tight for balance. Rest your head directly between your arms, and keep your chest open. Do not overstretch. It is not necessary to bend far, just at a slight angle from the body, so that you feel a stretch down the right side of your body. *Hold for three seconds*, then inhale and straighten up, lift back up onto your toes, then slowly lower the feet down, release the arms, and let them rest back at your sides. Take a full breath here and feel the difference between your left and right sides. Correct your posture, and inhale again slowly, raising the arms to the prayer position above your head, repeating the posture to the other side.

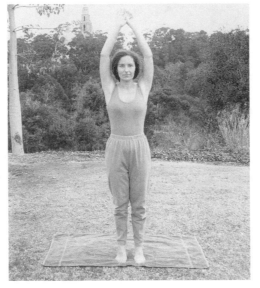

Half Moon Pose 1

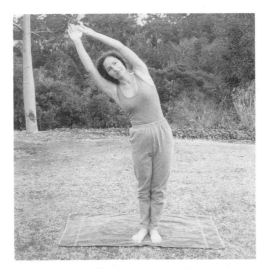

Half Moon Pose 2

Step 9: The Tree Pose

This balancing posture stretches the inner thighs and strengthens your arms and legs. In addition to these physical benefits, the Tree Pose has a balancing effect on your moods and emotions. Try this first next to a wall start to move away from the wall. Stand tall, with your left side facing a wall (the edge of a chair or couch will also work) with an arm's distance between you and the wall. Rest your left palm against the wall and spread your feet about an inch apart. Check to be sure your weight is distributed evenly. Turn your right foot out so that your right heel meets the arch of your left foot. Slowly bend your right leg and draw the foot up your left leg until your right foot reaches your left knee. Use your right hand to place your foot as high on your left thigh as possible. Raise your right arm to shoulder level for balance. When you are comfortable in this pose, remove your hand from the wall and bring both hands to prayer position at your chest. *Hold the posture for one to three full breaths, or as long as you are steady.* Repeat on the other side.

If you are unable to comfortably bring your foot up to the level of your opposite knee, just go as far as you can. If you are unable to balance when you leave the support of the wall or a piece of furniture, just stay where you are. My body relaxes to the point where I am able to balance myself only when I focus on a point on the wall in front of me.

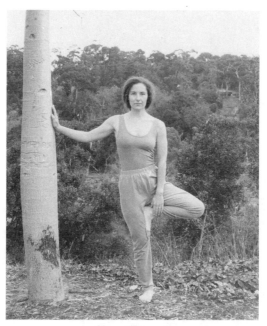

Tree Pose 1

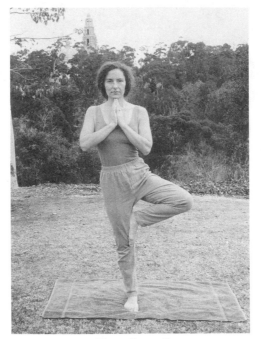

Tree Pose 2

Step 10: Spinal Twist

This pose stretches and strengthens the muscles in your back and stomach and firms the waist. This posture also aids digestion by providing gentle pressure to the digestive region. Sit on the floor with your right leg outstretched in front of you and your left leg bent, foot flat on the floor. Inhale deeply and sit up tall, elongating your spine. Rest your left hand behind you for balance and support and your right elbow against the outside of your left knee. Take another deep breath, and as you exhale, gently twist to the left. To increase the twist, press your elbow against your knee. *Hold this pose for three deep breaths, relaxing further into the twist on each exhalation.* Repeat on the other side.

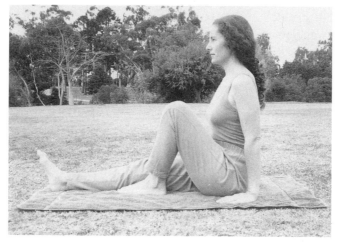

Spinal Twist 1

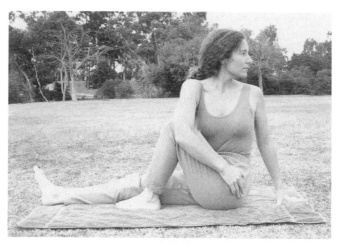

Spinal Twist 2

Step 11: Child's Pose

This final posture is for relaxing the whole body. In this pose you gather up all of the energy of the previous postures and focus on relaxing. Sit in a kneeling position on the ground. With your arms loose by your sides, slowly lower your chest to your knees, keeping your buttocks near your feet, as you rest on your calves. Let your forehead rest on the ground in front of your knees. Try not to let your buttocks raise too far off your feet. Let your arms rest loosely beside your legs, with your palms facing upward. Close your eyes and focus on your breath. *Take three full breaths*, slowly inhaling and exhaling, letting every muscle melt into the pose. Feel the energy flowing through your body, awakening and recharging every single cell. To come out of the pose, place your hands on your knees and slowly press yourself up, keeping your eyes closed and chin tucked until you are sitting straight up.

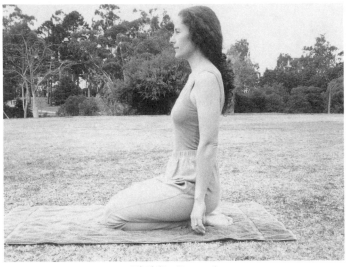

Child's Pose 1

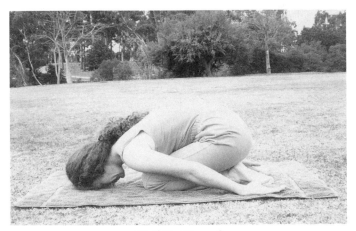

Child's Pose 2

As you become more comfortable in these postures, begin holding them longer and with greater concentration. The postures here are only a small sample of yoga poses, meant simply to get your spine moving and your body relaxing. There are a number of excellent books on yoga that you can consult for a more thorough approach. Or take a yoga class. If you do not know of any instructors in your area, ask a friend. Otherwise, check your phone directory or consult *Yoga Journal's* state-by-state directory of yoga teachers published each July.

EXERCISING THE BODY, ENERGIZING THE SOUL

Whether you choose to do yoga, take a walk, garden vigorously, any other form of exercise, or some combination of activities, the most important part of this Wellness Rx week is that you are consistent—every day and no less than twenty minutes a day. Remember, the twenty minutes can be spread out over the day. Take a ten-minute walk from work; run around with the kids for five minutes in the yard when you get home from work; do five minutes of yoga before you go to sleep. However, do the full routine of yoga exercises at least two times this week.

The important thing is that you give your body and especially your mind a chance to accept your new activity. Your ego may tell you at first that watching television before you go to bed will make you more relaxed than doing yoga. Remember, that is your ego talking, not your soul. But once you begin to incorporate exercise into your life, the soul's longing for energy and attention will overpower the ego's lazy habits.

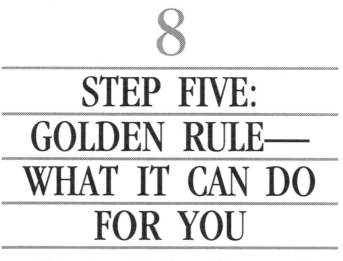

8

STEP FIVE: GOLDEN RULE— WHAT IT CAN DO FOR YOU

"I promise not to do anything wrong."

Goodness is medicine for your body, mind, and soul. Being a totally good person for the seven days of the Wellness Rx will have some very real effects on your health and energy. Most important, it will make you feel good about yourself. Your health is determined primarily by what you are willing to do for yourself. When you feel good about yourself, you are more willing to deepen your care for yourself and your soul.

Ethics and morals have become a complex topic these days because they have become so tangled up in politics and religious preferences. Jerry Falwell and the Dalai Lama speak about ethics and morals, but are they really talking about the same thing? My purpose is to reintroduce a very simple and elemental principle—a modern Golden Rule.

The Wellness Rx week is a spiritual and emotional timeout. It is a week to cultivate self-value, personal responsibility, and reverence for life, the framework for wellness. This is an opportunity to bring ethical awareness more centrally into every aspect of your life—eating, exercise, and your relations with others. This promise requires you to expand your consciousness of yourself as a good person more completely into your life.

It is not my intent to dictate to you what is "right" and what is "wrong." The only way to make these determinations is by truly listening to your soul. At some level, we are all struggling over what is right and what is wrong. However, during the week of the Wellness Rx, your task is to consciously intervene in this internal struggle by inserting a code of ethics that will determine your thinking and your behavior regarding yourself and others.

WE ARE SPIRITUAL BEINGS PRACTICING TO BE HUMAN

Moral values are instilled in you from birth. You usually know when you are doing something right versus something wrong. Your inner barometer makes you feel fine instead of apprehensive. It allows an inner smile instead of sweaty palms. Consider how lying to someone you love makes you feel. Then feel the difference between that feeling and a feeling of loving and honesty. Joy and peace come back to you when you are good.

You have all the goodness already in you that you will ever need. We are all souls bathed in starlight, connected one to another, like snowflakes joined in covering the mountaintops. By focusing on your inner strength as a spiritual being you know what is right and what is wrong. Can you imagine what might happen if all the spiritual beings began to blossom and join hands, covering the land like snowflakes?

Ethical living is a powerful antidote for illness. Indeed, the medical profession was founded on a sacred ethic, *primum non nocere*, "first, do no harm." This ethic of care need not apply solely to physicians. Since health is a spiritual discovery, it involves each of us and therefore requires that *primum non nocere* guide the personal practices of everyone—patients as well as doctors.

Don't you sometimes wonder whatever happened to the concept of sin? Ignoring the difference between right and wrong certainly has nothing to do with intelligence or wealth. Students at the Massachusetts Institute of Technology have brilliant intellects and pay astronomical tuitions, but a reported 83 percent of them recently admitted that they have cheated at least once in college.

Whether we do wrong by cheating, lying, stealing, littering, gossiping, or whatever else we might do, we *choose* to live with unnecessary burdens. Why should we make such a choice when it is possible for us to be kind, honest, decent, thoughtful, considerate, nonviolent individuals? Therefore, for the Wellness Rx week, promise to do nothing wrong. That means promising to do nothing that you even *think* might possibly be wrong.

HELPING OTHERS IS A POWERFUL HEALER

How do you know if something, some action or some word, is wrong? Some people describe feeling as though they were punched in the stomach. Others say they feel weak or momentarily confused. All of us have experienced how quickly our heart beats when we sense we are doing something wrong, and we are familiar with an uncomfortable feeling that also triggers an entire physiological response: body temperature rises, muscles tense, perspiration begins, and the whole body gears up to "fight or take flight." That feeling we have when we know we have not behaved correctly is a reliable inner guide to what is wrong. But this feeling goes beyond just a physical response. It is your soul, the center of your consciousness, that perpetually guides you toward right behavior and steers you from acts that are harmful to yourself or to others.

When the voice of the soul is hushed and the Healing Force is dim, our inner guide to what is right and wrong is difficult to perceive. Errors in judgment occur because we no longer hear that voice clearly amidst the din of mental clutter as we shuttle back and forth into the past and into the future, with our minds constantly straying from the present.

Only when we are calm and our minds are quiet can we turn within and listen to our inner guide. Our thoughts are moving so rapidly at times that it is no wonder we sometimes have difficulty discerning between right and wrong behavior. Too often our decisions to act in particular ways are made in haste, amidst the clutter and static in our minds, without proper reflection about the consequences of that action.

In line at the grocery store recently, I was standing behind a father with his two children. Their cart was piled high with groceries, and the children were clearly not satisfied with what had gone into the shopping cart. They tearfully protested what was missing: "Why not candy, Daddy? Mommy always buys us candy when she does the shopping." As their father sorted through his shopping list and his coupons, the frustration on his face was apparent. When his daughter, probably about four years old, handed, with pleading eyes, a sack of Hershey® bars to him, he snapped, "Do you have any idea how much it costs to feed this family every week? I don't care what you usually get at the store. Today, no Hershey® bars and no tears either. Period!" Of course, his daughter's eyes immediately welled up with tears, and it was clear how much he regretted his harsh response. He lifted his little girl up and apologized for snapping at her, explaining that he was very tired and frustrated and couldn't even find the coupons that her mother had asked him to take with him.

How often do we all snap at someone rather than thinking carefully about what we want to say and the effect it might have? When husbands and wives, parents and children, or friends and acquaintances snap at each other it means that one is suppressing the genuine feeling of the other and the other is merely crying out to be understood. When our emotions are raw, we are more likely to act or speak out of haste and without awareness of potential consequences, to ourselves or others. It is hard to "do the right thing" under these circumstances.

HOW TO FEEL GOOD ABOUT YOURSELF

When everything you do is done with peace and with your thoughts in the present, you will do no wrong. When you practice peacefulness, everything you do will have the effect of peace. The best way to ensure that you will behave kindly in response to the words or actions of another person is to make sure that everything you do is done with the peace of mind that comes from your thoughts being in the here and now.

You can be angry about the past only if your thoughts are in the past, and you can be worried about the future only if your thoughts are there too. By being attentive to where your thoughts are, it is possible to corral them and bring them back to the present moment. Your attentiveness is able to stop your thoughts from rambling around in yesterday or daydreaming in tomorrow. In this way, you can practice *peacefulness* in everything you do. Concentrate on keeping your thoughts in the present this week and you will practice the presence of peace and learn to live with the ethic of caring. Staying in the present will help protect you from wrongdoing and, in turn, will nurture your personal responsibility, self-value, and reverence for life.

Ahimsa is a beautiful Sanskrit word meaning "nonviolence." Ahimsa was the essence of all the goodness that Gandhi brought to India and the world. The same principle was the core of Martin Luther King, Jr.'s teachings and strategies for the establishment of civil rights in this country. My favorite example of practicing ahimsa is from a story about *le grande docteur*, Albert Schweitzer, as told by another man of exceptional ethical and moral caliber, the late Norman Cousins.

Dr. Schweitzer was receiving a visit at his medical hospital in Africa from Adlai Stevenson, the former presidential candidate. On a tour of the hospital compound, Stevenson suddenly stopped to swat a mosquito that had landed on Dr. Schweitzer's forearm. The doctor was taken aback, and although his response was "leavened with humor," his point was clear: "You shouldn't have done that. That was my mosquito and it wasn't necessary to call out the Sixth Fleet to deal with him."

The Great Doctor had a great sense of ethics, which his entire life exemplified. Schweitzer lived by an ethic of care that says, "First, do no harm," in his relations with all living things. In this he included plants, animals, and insects, as well as his fellow human beings and the planet they inhabit. "We are ethical," said Schweitzer, "only when life, as such, is sacred." It may be too difficult to live entirely up to Doctor Schweitzer's standards, but we can still take the time not to litter our environment, and when we remove a daddy-longlegs or spider from our living-room wall, we can place it gently on the ground outside.

Your inner strength and morality are the very source of your being. This week will cause you to focus on your very source. Following the Golden Rule will allow you to touch that source. Take care to make each moment of this Wellness Rx week sacred and free of selfishness. Radiant health that is grounded in your soul and expands outward cannot be cultivated without actively pursuing a moral life. The simplest and highest form of moral living is to cultivate a sense of reverence for and connection with all life. Listen to the inner guide of your soul. And above all, first, do no wrong.

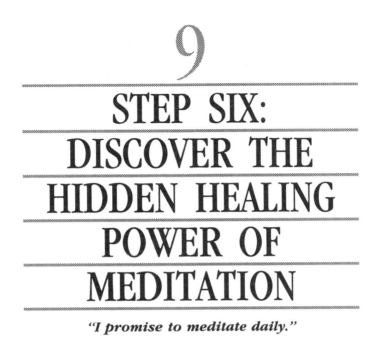

9

STEP SIX: DISCOVER THE HIDDEN HEALING POWER OF MEDITATION

"I promise to meditate daily."

Everything you do should be done with peace. That is the best medicine for your body, mind, and soul.
—*Paramahansa Yogananda*

Unless you have previously visited a practitioner of alternative medical systems, such as Ayurveda or Chinese medicine, chances are high that no traditional Western physician has ever written you a prescription for meditation. In my own clinical experience, however, I have come to learn that the most potent prescription I can recommend to any patient is not a pharmaceutical medication but a healthy dose of meditation. The main ingredients in a life filled with radiant health and energy are peace, balance, and energy. Meditation promotes all three.

If our souls are like compasses with a needle pointing us back toward our "soul" purpose, which is love and wellness, then our minds are like the winds of a fierce storm that blow us off course. When those winds are calmed and our minds are fresh like the crisp blue sky following a storm, our inner compass is direct and our purpose is clear. In those moments we experience great health and happiness, and we feel alive with energy and strength.

What we need, then, is a technique for calming those mental storms. Meditation is the process of taking hold of the mind and pulling it back into the present. It is the practice of consciously quieting all of the disturbing mental chatter; clearing away the cobwebs of thoughts, worries, and fears; and uncovering the source of all clarity and peace within us. Meditation quiets the mind and strengthens the soul. When we meditate, we are literally ensouled, surrounded by the healing glow that the soul exudes when it is allowed to sing. In meditation we taste the vital joy that has been suppressed by negative emotions and thoughts. Experiencing that joy is the key to cultivating better health.

For the seven days of the Wellness Rx, promise yourself that you will meditate daily. Dispel any preconceived negative notions you have about meditation and think of it simply as *learning to practice the presence of peace.* The meditation exercise I will describe shortly is not tied to any particular religion and is perfectly compatible with whatever spiritual beliefs you embrace. If you want to plant the seeds of wellness within, you have to uproot the weeds of thought nestled in your mind that are contributing to your stress and illness. Meditation is the key to unlocking wellness.

How to Experience Joy and Peace

Meditation is the practice of bringing your mind into the moment. Only when your mind is present in the moment can you pass through the gateway to your soul and experience the peace that resides within. That peace is the heart of the universe, the source of all life, and it dwells within every human being. The most direct way to establish that connection, to restore that peace within, is to dive deep beneath the clouds of thought, emotion, and desire to the deepest levels of your consciousness, the inner light of your soul.

Nearly all cultures and religions of the world have some tradition of meditation. The great teachers of these cultural traditions have proclaimed in strikingly similar fashion that within every separate individual is an immortal soul that connects us all with the infinite. In Christianity it is declared, "The Kingdom of Heaven is within." Ancient Buddhist teachings instruct, "If you wish to seek the Buddha, you ought to see into your own Nature for this Nature is the Buddha himself." Siddhartha echoed this thought when he said, "One must find the source within one's own Self; one must possess it." An American Indian spiritual song rejoices, "It is there that our hearts are set, in the expanse of the heavens." "Do not search in distant skies for God," says

Shintoism. "In man's own heart is He found." And Jesus proclaimed in the Sermon on the Mount, "You are the light of the world." All great teachers have taught this same universal truth.

These lessons are registered in some of the world's most beloved and admired artists and poets. The famous Italian musician Puccini declared that the secret of all creative geniuses is that they are attuned to the beauty, grandeur, and sublimity within their own souls, "which are part of Omnipotence," and that they share this beauty with others.

The poet Robert Browning conveyed the same sentiments in his poem named for the ancient physician, Paracelsus:

> *There is an inmost center in us all,*
> *Where truth abides in fullness; and around,*
> *Wall upon wall, the gross flesh hems it in,*
> *This perfect, clear perception—which is truth.*

Meditation is the practice of diving down into that innermost center where truth resides, uncluttered and undiluted by harmful thoughts, emotions, beliefs, and attitudes. Meditation opens up a doorway to the soul where we can experience the stillness and calm that inspire total wellness.

A Spiritual Spring Cleaning

The poet William Blake wrote of the mind: "If the doors of perception were cleansed, everything would be seen as it is, infinite." For most of us, our minds presently work in overdrive, darting here, darting there, constantly navigating between recollections of the past and anticipations of the future. Our doors of perception are obstructed by a tall heap of thoughts, worries, fears, anxieties, angers, frustrations, beliefs, and attitudes that will not budge on their own accord. If we hope to open those doors of perception, to clear away the debris that shuts out the clarity lying behind those doors, we must begin a spiritual spring cleaning.

The promises and practices of the Wellness Rx are the "cleaning supplies" that can accomplish the task that Blake sets before us. Meditation is a key phase of this cleaning. Without neutralizing the negative thoughts and emotions that contribute to our illnesses, achieved through the process of meditation, all we are doing is something like sweeping dust under the rug. The thoughts and feelings and attitudes are swept away where no one can see them. But the important thing is that you know they are still there. Meditation is the instrument that reaches into the crevices of your mind where harmful thoughts are buried and uproots them. When the doors of perception are cleared away, they will open up to reveal the inner truth that resides in the soul.

While spiritual teachers have long recognized the importance of various forms of meditation for nourishing the soul, medical researchers have recently begun to explore the health benefits of meditation and relaxation. The Wellness Rx embraces both emphases and suggests, indeed, that the spiritual and medical benefits of meditation are deeply connected.

Meditation has been scientifically proven to eliminate or reverse many illnesses and diseases brought on by harmful responses to stress. The technique of meditation presented here is entirely compatible with and will enhance the effects of traditional approaches to medicine. Hundreds of scientific studies have investigated the physiological effects of meditation. Most provide evidence that shows that meditation lowers respiration, reduces oxygen consumption, and slows the rate of metabolism. The relaxation that accompanies meditation has also been demonstrated to slow the pulse, ease tension in the muscles, and slow the manufacture of adrenaline and other potentially harmful chemicals. Studies have further shown that during meditation the activity of the brain slows, as evidenced by an increase in low-frequency alpha, theta and delta waves, which are those brain activities associated with relaxation.

You can coax your mind into calmness the same way you can train your muscles to stretch and strengthen. It is there, in that state of calmness, that inner peace is born and nurtured. In meditation you are at peace with your body and your mind. You are even at peace with your illnesses. Now, I do not mean that you like whatever illness ails you, and I am not suggesting that you "make illness your friend." What I am saying, however, is that your best strategy for defusing illness is to strengthen your soul's healing resources.

PREPARING YOURSELF FOR LASTING HEALING

Stand up and tackle your illnesses, but do it with peace. Responses to illness driven by guilt, anger, fear, or bitterness have only temporary effects. Peace is a permanent medicine. When you respond to illness with peace, you prepare yourself for lasting healing.

Worry and fear about illness only compound your pain. When you meditate, your awareness of your bodily pain or discomfort melts away into your awareness of your life as so much larger than your physical body. Because meditation makes you aware of how much more you are than just this body, it is a sanctuary of silence that no disease can invade. In a spiritual letter, St. John of the Cross wrote that "whereas speaking distracts, silence and action collect the thoughts, and strengthen the spirit." All diseases are weak beside a strong spirit.

Meditation fans the flame of the Healing Force, which the Wellness Rx helps you reignite. Meditation takes us into the center of our self, into the soul, that St. Teresa referred to as the "Interior Castle." Once we step inside that castle, we listen quietly to the inner song of our soul. This is the greatest protection against all disease.

Remember that illness is an imbalance in the body's perfect energy. The practice of daily meditation restores inner balance and allows healing energy to be directed where it is needed. Meditation is not a substitute for standard medicinal treatments. But while medication targets a specific symptom, meditation heals by going straight to the deeper source of illness. Whereas medication is aimed at a particular site of the body, meditation reverberates throughout every cell and has a global healing influence.

Every cell, every muscle, every ounce of your being responds to even a few moments of silent meditation. These periods of quiet inward reflection unleash the flow of healing energy from your soul. Illnesses, aches, infections, and other physical ailments are the obstacles to this flow of healing energy. Meditation brings you to a level beyond your physical discomforts, even beyond the harmful or negative thoughts percolating in your mind. When you sit quietly in meditation, you sit in the presence of your soul. There, you sit in the presence of peace.

YOUR DAILY MEDITATION PROGRAM

I am going to teach you a way to meditate that I worked out with over 1,000 children before I went on to teach it successfully to over 50,000 adults. If children as young as three or four years old and adults as old as ninety-five are able to do this meditation, surely you will be able to do it too.

This meditation exercise will open wide the doors to healing and radiant health. The exercise described is certainly not the only form of meditation. You may already be practicing some type of meditation. If your method feels comfortable and you are able to quiet your mind using those techniques, then continue with them. The most important thing about meditation is that it feels right for you. You can tailor the exercises here to correspond with your own spiritual or religious beliefs. If you feel a strong bond with nature, make your meditation a time to focus on that connection. If you are devoted to a particular saint, hold his or her image in your mind when you meditate. Or you may feel drawn to a certain sacred word— *amen, shalom, om, peace,* or *love.* You may find it calming to hold this word in your mind, repeating it inwardly and in silence.

Whatever form of meditation you choose, you will need a comfortable, quiet place. In the warm months, I like to sit outside in the sunshine, beneath the tree in my backyard. When it becomes too cold for meditating outside, I move to a comfortable and warm place indoors, in my bedroom, or in front of the fireplace. Wear loose clothes, such as sweat pants, so that you can sit comfortably, on the floor or in a chair. Sit up tall and with good posture. If you are sitting on the floor, place a firm pillow beneath you. Try to shut out all distractions. Turn off the ringer to the phone and let the answering machine pick it up, and ask others around you to allow you ten or twenty minutes alone. If there is noise you cannot control, a lawnmower outside or children playing, play some gentle music quietly in the background. How long you meditate is up to you and will depend on how much time you can set aside. For the Wellness Rx week, insist upon at least seven minutes a day, a length that even the busiest person can stick to. Eventually your meditation time will increase as you learn to dive deep into your awareness.

Meditation Technique
Practicing the Presence of Peace

- Close your eyes and consciously relax your breathing. Breathe naturally, through your nose, and with each breath draw in a feeling of peace and calm.
- Now, take a long, even, relaxed breath, and as you exhale relax your forehead and the muscles behind your eyes.
- Take a long, even, relaxed breath, and as you exhale release the tension around your mouth, jaw, and neck.
- Take a long, even, relaxed breath, and as you exhale relax your shoulders, arms, hands, and fingers.

- Take a long, even, relaxed breath, and as you exhale let go of the tension in your chest and abdomen.

- Take a long, even, relaxed breath, and as you exhale relax the muscles throughout your back and buttocks.

- Take a long, even, relaxed breath, and as you exhale release the tension in your thighs, calves, feet, and toes.

- Take a long, even, relaxed breath, and as you exhale picture a radiant golden healing light filling your entire body from your toes to the very tip of your head.

- Continue to breathe slowly and deeply and inwardly affirm over and over to yourself: I am loved . . . I am loved . . . I am loved . . . I am loved . . . I am loved.

- Continue repeating this for as long as you wish. Before finishing, sit quietly for a moment, eyes closed, feeling the presence of peace permeating every cell of your body.

CASE HISTORY—HELP BANISH ARTHRITIS WITH MEDITATION

Peter was a fifty-seven-year-old patient who came to me because he had severe pain accompanying arthritis in his knees and ankles. His legs were so gripped by pain that just walking from the parking lot to my examination room made Peter tearful. When he sat in the chair across from my desk, I could see he was still in enormous pain as he rubbed the muscles around his knees. Seeing his pain made my own heart ache, and there was nothing more that I wanted in that moment than to give him some relief, a few moments without the needles and pins piercing through his legs.

After introductions, I asked Peter to let me do something for him that might seem unusual. "If you've got something to ease this pain, I'll take whatever it is." Peter was expecting medication, not meditation, but I asked him to sit as comfortably as he could and close his eyes. I guided him through the basic meditation described above for just five minutes. When we came to the final section, where "I am loved . . . I am loved. . . . " is repeated inwardly, I asked Peter to continue as long as he felt comfortable, and to open his eyes when he was ready.

Twenty minutes later, Peter opened his eyes with an expression of alertness and amazement. "I have to tell you this. My legs don't ache at all, and they ached like hell up until just now." Peter had no idea how much time had passed and was embarrassed that I might think he had fallen asleep during our visit. Meditation is different from sleeping, though. During meditation your mind is alert, and you are very much awake. Peter's experience is a common one. Having never experienced the calmness of meditation, he was easily absorbed into it. Because his mind was so focused in the moment, following his breath, he lost track of time.

Peter still has arthritis in his legs, but he is no longer controlled by the pain. Meditating regularly, he is now able to control and calm his mental chatter and direct his awareness soulward rather than focusing every ounce of his energy on the pain in his legs. You can use the same process to alleviate the discomfort of any illness or disease. Whether you are currently sick or basically healthy, this simple practice of meditation will instill a greater sense of peace in your life. This peace is the greatest source of limitless freedom.

10

STEP SEVEN: BE
HAPPY, NOT RIGHT

*"I promise to adopt the philosophy that it is more important
to be happy than right."*

I was a child during the Second World War, growing up in a neighborhood of diverse cultures in the Bronx. Being Jewish made my brother and me targets of frequent hostility and sometimes physical violence delivered by other children too young to really understand the meaning of their actions. One afternoon on the way home from school, my brother and I were chased by a group of boys wielding wooden sticks. We made our way through narrow alleys and up fire escapes to our tiny apartment, where our mother was busy working. Adrenaline rushing, blood pumping, we described the scene to our mother while we tore through the closets looking for anything with which to protect ourselves.

What my mother told me that afternoon has stuck with me all of my life: "Anyone can fight back. But it really takes a courageous person to forgive. Only forgiveness can conquer hatred."

Harbored deep in our minds and hearts are all of the sadnesses, all of the hurts, the angers, frustrations, disappointments, and betrayals gathered up over the years that we have never forgiven. The burdens of unforgiven angers and hurts that we carry around with us are like tight knots in the fabric of our being. Although we may rarely recall these memories, they are like rocks we have to climb over to reach the peace of our inner cathedral.

How Forgiveness Leads to Healing

The effects these emotional burdens have on health can no longer be ignored. The knots of unresolved disputes, unforgiven acts, and unkind words are distributed throughout the body, where they impede the healing flow of life energy and create the conditions for disease. They clog arteries, stiffen joints, tighten muscles, raise the pulse, burn into ulcers, and grip the heart. There is clear scientific evidence that these thoughts, feelings, emotions, and memories influence the balance of health and illness in our lives.

By adopting the philosophy that *it is more important to be happy than right* during the Wellness Rx week, you begin to untie the knots of past hurts, angers, and disappointments that are influencing your energy and balance. When you make the promise to choose happiness over being right, you effectively promise to no longer erect the emotional barricades to radiant health and energy.

Ninety-nine percent of the things we fight about and insist we are right about, on a daily basis, are just worthless. Who forgot to turn off the light, who was late, who dirtied the carpet, who was supposed to call but forgot—the daily struggles we engage in with our spouse, parent, child, friend, coworkers, grocery clerk, and others are in the grand scheme of things just unimportant, and yet they do so much damage to our well-being.

I am not asking you to betray your deepest beliefs or disregard your principles. I am not suggesting that you compromise your integrity in the face of conflict by putting on a smile instead of standing up for what you believe. Nor am I recommending that you live your life trying to please everyone at the risk of being untrue to yourself.

What I am asking you to become aware of, however, is how often we engage in fights that are less over higher principles and a deep sense of personal integrity and more about, simply, being right. In the larger picture, how important is it, really, to be right about who left the light on? What does it matter, in the greater scheme of your life, that you get to be right in a conflict over who provoked a particular disagreement? In such matters it is not the soul that aspires to be right, it is the ego. At those moments you would do well to keep in mind that it is your ego that has probably backed you into this situation in the first place and is probably not the most reliable source of getting you out of it.

The next time you become embroiled in a conflict, recognize that it is only important to your ego that you are right. It is your ego, not the other person, with which you are fighting. By accepting happiness over being right, you disarm the ego's power over you, and ultimately, your health. Arguing, disagreeing, or haggling about where to place blame will never end a fight. Remember the old saying, "It takes two to tango." When you refuse to participate in a battle, the battle no longer exists. When you accept that it is more important to be happy than right, you can no longer be swept up in the unhealthy dance of anger.

Avoiding Meaningless Conflict

Conflicts are not meaningful unless you attribute meaning to them. If what you are arguing about has nothing to do with your soul purpose, then it has no meaning and is not worth investing with meaning. During the Wellness Rx week, if you find yourself engaging in a struggle or confrontation with another person, recognize that at a much more important level, you are fighting with yourself. Peace is your natural state. You were born in peace and an infinite source of peace resides always within you. Anything that denies or assaults this peace is against your nature and is not worthy of your investment.

If someone treats you unkindly or with anger, pay attention to your inner peace. There is no greater way to conquer hostility or unkindness than with forgiveness and peace. Returning unkind words with verbal barbs and daggers only makes the "hot water" you are in hotter. Have you ever tried to quarrel with someone who will not respond? Do you know how hard it is to be unkind to someone who is nothing but kind to you? When you can learn to return unkindness with kindness, anger with joy, and hostility with peace, you will know happiness and how to inspire it in others, even—especially—those whom you find it hard to call "friend."

Arguments are like snowballs. The more snow you pile up on top of them, the faster they roll. Have you ever reached the point in an argument where it just seems out of control? Harsh words are flying, accusations are slinging, and at some point, the argument seems to have taken on a life of its own. In a sense, it has, because you have poured so much of your life energy into giving this argument meaning. That is why arguments wear you out. All of the energy you invest in being right, all of the life you pour into the argument, strips you of vital energy. To stay alive, arguments need to take the life out of us.

If someone is shouting at you, throwing hurtful words your way, tune out those words and focus on hearing the inner voice of your soul. Your ego will tell you to fight back, shout out, and will even provide you the hateful words to dish it out. But if you can shut out those thoughts and reflect back on your inner voice, your soul will tell you to forgive and be peaceful. With practice, soon you will find that in the face of confrontation, your mind will not be filled with harmful words to sling, because you have replaced those thoughts with the compelling force of love and kindness that is the voice of your soul.

Just as an angry response fuels the fires of conflict and hatred, a peaceful response generates peace and kindness. "A joy shared," wrote Goethe, "is a joy doubled." Let the anger in others inspire you to make your life an example of joy. Do not try to change other people's behaviors. This is fruitless. Instead, change yourself, and by doing so you will positively affect others. If you want others to treat you with more kindness, be more kind yourself.

How easily we excuse our own faults. During the Wellness Rx week, actively practice forgiving others of their faults. The sacred texts of all religions teach forgiveness as a principle of spiritual, compassionate living. Forgiveness is a spiritual process because it requires that we be in touch with our higher—what I have been calling "soul"–purpose. It is our egos that drive us to stubbornly cling to old hurts and angers. Stubbornness is the language of the ego; the soul prefers forgiveness. The soul prefers forgiveness because to forgive is to act out of unselfish love. The *Mahabharata*, a great epic spiritual drama of India, instructs, "One should forgive, under any injury." In Judaism it is taught "the most beautiful thing a man can do is to forgive wrong."

HELP HEAL THE MOST COMMON HEALTH PROBLEMS WITH FORGIVENESS

The Wellness Rx asks that you forgive others at least seven times as frequently as you ask others to forgive you. If you find that you are unable to forgive the people you feel have caused you pain or hurt, take a long look at that inability. Confronting your hesitation to forgive others is like staring the source of your illnesses right in the face. You may be ill, experiencing arthritis, ulcers, migraine, insomnia, panic, hypertension, backache or obesity because you are burdened by all of the emotions you refuse to forgive. Forgiveness goes a long way in freeing you from disease because it breaks a vital link in the gripping chain of the past.

Do not be trapped by your anger, frustration, hurt, or worry. Part of living in the present moment requires forgiveness, because the unwillingness to forgive keeps you chained to the past. Grudges are not just mental attitudes living deep in the back of your mind. The grudges you hold against others are the back spasms, the ulcers, the tension headaches, the fatigue, the anxiety, the colitis, and all of the other physical symptoms that cause you discomfort and pain. You cannot simultaneously live in peace and nurture a longstanding grudge.

Being happy instead of right is not a sign of weakness or acquiescence. It takes a strong person to neutralize the ego's desires for self-gratification. Forgiveness requires tremendous strength, but it also generates strong improvements in your health and energy. If you find yourself in a potentially heated conversation or situation, resolve to neither agree nor disagree with the other party. Do not attach to anything spoken the labels "right" or "wrong." Instead, recognize the goodness in the other person, despite what they may be saying at the moment. Instead of judging that person, accept them as they are, another soul on a long journey home to God. When you learn to see and honor in others what is most hidden, what you most want to reveal in yourself, the difference between being happy instead of right will make perfect sense. When you recognize the unity between all souls to all things, it makes no sense to distinguish between "right" and "wrong."

Transcending the desire to always be "right," transcending the instinct to judge, are the greatest keys to soul happiness. The Wellness Rx will help you establish forgiveness as a mental blueprint or pattern of thought and action in your life. Combined with the healing power of unconditional love and an awareness of peace, the Wellness Rx will help you nurture the unmatchable source of healing kindling within you.

Never think that your individual acts of kindness and forgiveness have no effect. Every simple act of forgiving, every sincere smile, reverberates throughout yourself and those around you. When all is said and done, angry thoughts and hurt feelings will always be overcome by goodness, joy, and happiness.

11

PROCLAMATION FOR RADIANT HEALTH & ENERGY

This is the final and most crucial ingredient in the prescription. You have now learned the seven steps that will usher you across the bridge to wellness in seven days. However, before you begin your Wellness Rx, there is this final requirement: creating a personal proclamation to reclaim your health destiny.

This personal proclamation, in which you sign your name to a list of the seven promises outlined in the seven chapters preceding this, is crucial to your journey to wellness. It is like tying your shoelaces before you take a walk. You don't want to trip. By signing your name to this proclamation you personalize these promises and give them meaning in the context of your own life.

But signing the proclamation is more than just a "safeguard" against tripping across the bridge to wellness. Adding your signature to the seven Wellness Rx promises makes this prescription sacred. Your signature transforms a simple promise into sacred vows invested with all of your heart and soul.

You will now truly identify who you are. And what you are is a child of humanity created in the image of a much Higher Power. Live up to that image in every way. Walk with your head held up high, your heart open to love, your spirits soaring, and believe in yourself.

So now, take the first and most important step on your journey to wellness. Add your signature to the Wellness Rx promises and know that you are in charge of your own health destiny.

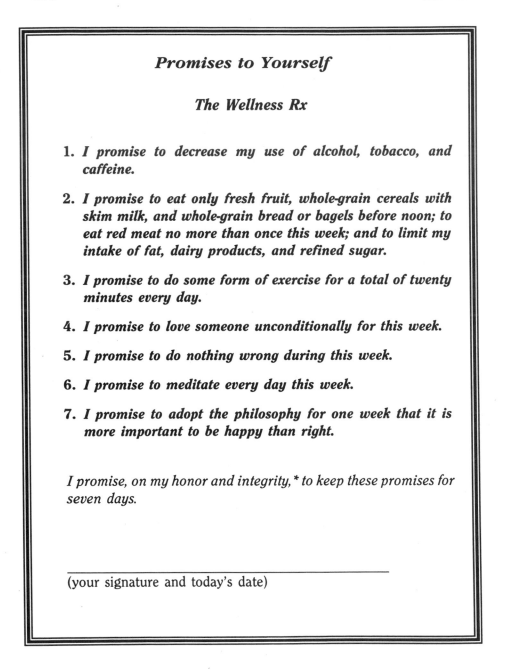

Promises to Yourself

The Wellness Rx

1. *I promise to decrease my use of alcohol, tobacco, and caffeine.*

2. *I promise to eat only fresh fruit, whole-grain cereals with skim milk, and whole-grain bread or bagels before noon; to eat red meat no more than once this week; and to limit my intake of fat, dairy products, and refined sugar.*

3. *I promise to do some form of exercise for a total of twenty minutes every day.*

4. *I promise to love someone unconditionally for this week.*

5. *I promise to do nothing wrong during this week.*

6. *I promise to meditate every day this week.*

7. *I promise to adopt the philosophy for one week that it is more important to be happy than right.*

I promise, on my honor and integrity,* to keep these promises for seven days.

_____

(your signature and today's date)

---

*Many of my patients have found it powerful to add "and I swear to God."

Congratulations! Signing your proclamation starts you well on your way to wellness, radiant health, and vibrant energy! Make a copy of your proclamation and place it somewhere visible to you, on your bedside dresser, your refrigerator door, or a bulletin board. Put your proclamation anywhere you will be likely to see it regularly. It will be a powerful reminder of the steps you are taking to reclaim your health destiny.

How to Keep Track of Your Wellness Rx

It is absolutely crucial that you keep records of your compliance with your own promises. On the following pages you will find a record-keeping system that consists of a day-to-day log and a week-at-a-glance calendar.

Simply check off each ingredient of the Wellness Rx as you accomplish it for that day. Also check it on the weekly calendar. I can absolutely assure you that you will feel better than you can possibly conceive of if you will just follow your own simple personal promises perfectly for seven days.

Remember, this is a prescription! You cannot decide to leave out any ingredients and you must follow it for seven days.

I strongly suggest that you carefully read through the stories of depression, insomnia, addiction, and physical pain in the next chapters. There will be a great deal of important information for you in these chapters even if you are not experiencing the particular problem being described.

YOUR DAILY RECORD OF PROMISES KEPT

MONDAY	TUESDAY	WEDNESDAY	THURSDAY	FRIDAY	SATURDAY	SUNDAY
1. Addiction ☐✔	1. ☐✔	1. ☐✔	1. ☐✔	1. ☐✔	1. ☐✔	1. ☐✔
2. Nutrition ☐✔	2. ☐✔	2. ☐✔	2. ☐✔	2. ☐✔	2. ☐✔	2. ☐✔
3. Exercise ☐✔	3. ☐✔	3. ☐✔	3. ☐✔	3. ☐✔	3. ☐✔	3. ☐✔
4. Lovingness ☐✔	4. ☐✔	4. ☐✔	4. ☐✔	4. ☐✔	4. ☐✔	4. ☐✔
5. Golden Rule ☐✔	5. ☐✔	5. ☐✔	5. ☐✔	5. ☐✔	5. ☐✔	5. ☐✔
6. Meditation ☐✔	6. ☐✔	6. ☐✔	6. ☐✔	6. ☐✔	6. ☐✔	6. ☐✔
7. Happy, Not Right ☐✔	7. ☐✔	7. ☐✔	7. ☐✔	7. ☐✔	7. ☐✔	7. ☐✔
PROMISES	*PROMISES*	*PROMISES*	*PROMISES*	*PROMISES*	*PROMISES*	*PROMISES*

MONDAY

1. I am dealing with my addictions

_____ ☐✓

2. I am following my nutrition promise

_____ ☐✓

3. I have exercised or practiced yoga

_____ ☐✓

4. I have loved (write in name) unconditionally

_____ ☐✓

5. I have done nothing wrong

_____ ☐✓

6. I have meditated

_____ ☐✓

7. I have chosen to be happy rather than right

_____ ☐✓

TUESDAY

1. Addiction— _____

   _____

   _____ □✓

2. Nutrition— _____

   _____

   _____ □✓

3. Exercise— _____

   _____

   _____ □✓

4. Lovingness— _____

   _____

   _____ □✓

5. Golden Rule— _____

   _____

   _____ □✓

6. Meditation— _____

   _____

   _____ □✓

7. Happy, not right— _____

   _____

   _____ □✓

WEDNESDAY

1. _____

   _____

   _____ □✓

2. _____

   _____

   _____ □✓

3. _____

   _____

   _____ □✓

4. _____

   _____

   _____ □✓

5. _____

   _____

   _____ □✓

6. _____

   _____

   _____ □✓

7. _____

   _____

   _____ □✓

THURSDAY

I. _____

_____

_____ ☐✔

2. _____

_____

_____ ☐✔

3. _____

_____

_____ ☐✔

4. _____

_____

_____ ☐✔

5. _____

_____

_____ ☐✔

6. _____

_____

_____ ☐✔

7. _____

_____

_____ ☐✔

FRIDAY

1. _____
   _____
   _____ ☐✔

2. _____
   _____
   _____ ☐✔

3. _____
   _____
   _____ ☐✔

4. _____
   _____
   _____ ☐✔

5. _____
   _____
   _____ ☐✔

6. _____
   _____
   _____ ☐✔

7. _____
   _____
   _____ ☐✔

SATURDAY

I. _____
_____
_____ ☐✓

2. _____
_____
_____ ☐✓

3. _____
_____
_____ ☐✓

4. _____
_____
_____ ☐✓

5. _____
_____
_____ ☐✓

6. _____
_____
_____ ☐✓

7. _____
_____
_____ ☐✓

SUNDAY

1. _____
   _____
   _____ ☐✓

2. _____
   _____
   _____ ☐✓

3. _____
   _____
   _____ ☐✓

4. _____
   _____
   _____ ☐✓

5. _____
   _____
   _____ ☐✓

6. _____
   _____
   _____ ☐✓

7. _____
   _____
   _____ ☐✓

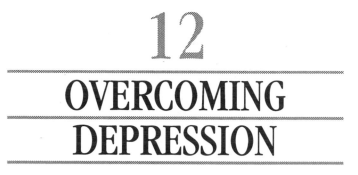

OVERCOMING DEPRESSION

Truly it is in the darkness that one finds the light, so when we are in sorrow, then this light is nearest of all to us.

—*Meister Eckhart*

Depression confronts medical science with a fundamental problem. Feelings of worthlessness, despair, helplessness, and loneliness typically cause a multitude of physical symptoms, including arthritis, fatigue, hypertension, headache, backache, digestive problems, and general pains. But in most cases, depression is not caused by a physical condition. Depression is generally the manifestation of unresolved emotional, psychological, social, or spiritual burdens. Given no outlet, these burdens weigh down the body, mind, and heart. The problem for medicine is that our most common treatments for depression—antidepressant prescription drugs—don't provide ultimate remedies because they just don't access the ultimate source of the depression. Indeed, potent drugs may create an even greater distance between the person and the source of his or her depression because they numb rather than uproot the hidden pain.

CASE HISTORY—JOHN WILLIAMS STRUGGLES WITH JEALOUSY AND HIS PAST

I met a patient named John Williams last year. He had been severely depressed for many months, despite a number of different antidepressant medications. Indeed, John came to me because he felt the antidepressants were just making matters worse, polishing up the outside but leaving his "inside works" in a mess. We agreed that any solution to his depression would lie in personal strategies for melting the hurts and angers that were frozen within him like a river in the heart of winter. I watched this man as he learned to chip away at that frozen block of accumulated pains, hardened prejudices, sad memories, and failed expectations.

In less than one week I saw remarkable changes in the patient's level of energy, outlook, and physical appearance. Most of all, I heard in his voice the growing sense of value and self-worth that this man had been seeking for years in all of the wrong places. Looking inside himself, far beneath an armor of toughness and false strength he erected over the years, he found self-value, personal responsibility, and reverence for life, and it was there that he found the cure for his depression.

Depression is an ailment of the soul. It is the expression of energy stopped dead in its tracks, frozen solid. What overcoming depression requires, then, is a cleansing of the pathways of energy in the mind, body, and soul. Depression is the absence of vitality, an obstruction in the flow of your life energy. This obstruction can be removed, cleared away to make room for ever-new energy and boundless vitality. But medicine alone will not accomplish this task. Only a soulful approach, a spiritual spring cleaning, can remedy a soul sickness. It requires searching through the darkness that surrounds you in your depression and reaching for even the tiniest flickering of light that burns eternal in all souls.

The following pages chronicle John's search for a way out of the darkness of his depression. With the patient's kind permission, I have chosen to reveal a substantial amount of our private interaction because this individual drowning in a river of despair, in spite of swimming harder and harder, could be any one of us. Whatever the specific nature of your depression or despair, a similar process of turning up the light in your soul is necessary if you want to leave such darkness behind forever. John Williams brought me close to that darkness, and there I saw how close to the eternal light of the Healing Force we all really are.

The story you are about to read is a fable for every person raised in a manner that interferes with his or her experience of happiness. The moral of the story is that it is no longer necessary to continue to live your parents' lives.

You can do much more than you think you can do. You can behave better than the way you were taught to behave, you can be more loving than you were brought up to be, you can accomplish more than you ever thought you could, and most important, you can make a plan to emerge from your most dire difficulties and sorrow through an infusion of radiant energy and hope.

Depression and anxiety are rampant these days, with more and more people plunging into depths of despair. Over 50 percent of the illnesses I treat are associated with episodes of sadness and sorrow. Patients are awash in torrents of tranquilizers and antidepressant medications, and some are even using Prozac merely to improve their normal personalities. Drugs may be useful, but the problem begins in the mind and the soul is pleading for help.

Meet John Williams now. He is middle aged and lives in the country, and he is surely an amazing character. As you listen to this person trapped in his own pain and locked into his own way of thinking, imagine him to be *your* age and sex and put him in the city if you wish. Then observe the struggle of a soul seeking love and warmth and follow its progress as a current of energy ignites and unleashes the power of the Healing Force.

Our First Meeting: Melting a Frozen River of Despair

We are healed from suffering only by experiencing it to the full.
—Marcel Proust

Patient: If I let myself, I could sleep forever. I'm so sad and blue, I could cry all the time.

Physician: When did this start?

Patient: When my wife and I had a problem and I thought it was serious and I was ready for a divorce. I wasn't really ready for a divorce, but I was going to get a divorce because I thought that was the only way I could retaliate. I am not sure what the right words are for it because I'm not very good at my vocabulary. I'm just a country boy and about all I know how to do is work. I am very particular in my work, and whatever I do, I try to do as good as the best or better. I am constantly wanting to do better, but I didn't know how to get better at my marriage.

My wife talked me into going to a doctor, and I decided to see a psychiatrist because I didn't want to bring this up with our family doctor. I guess I thought I was crazy. Anyway, the doctor suggested that I take some Prozac for depression. I started the pills, and I took them for three or four months and they seemed to be doing fine, except it affected my sexual ability drastically. I mentioned that to the doctor and he changed me to another pill. The new pills made me sleep all night and all day, and then all night again. I just skipped a day of chores and work completely. I called the doctor to tell him about that, and then I just stopped taking the pills. The pills didn't help me one bit on the inside. I'm not an old chair that you can just slap a new coat of paint on.

Physician: You said something before about needing to "retaliate." Against what?

Patient: I thought my wife had a fellow. I saw this stable hand coming on to my wife, severely. I am sorry, but I just can't tolerate that. So I saw this guy putting the moves on her, and I told her she needed to tell him to hit the bricks, but she wouldn't do that. So I did. She said I was just imagining things. Well, that didn't satisfy me. I really thought there was something there or she would have told the jerk to get lost.

Physician: So, was there something there?

Patient: Apparently not. I never saw my wife go after him, but I sure saw him come on to her. He is a drunken, no-good sop who doesn't own a damn thing at all. Her life with me is ten times better than he could give her.

Physician: So, is that why your depression began?

Patient: That's sure the stone that broke off the wagon wheel.

Physician: Were you doing fine before then?

Patient: I have never done fine, really. It is hard for people to live up to my expectations.

Physician: What does that mean?

Patient: I raise horses to sell at auctions. I work hard all the time and I'm working even harder now. You don't get very far by doing things just half way, you know?

Physician: I asked you when you were fine and you said you had never been fine. What does that mean?

Patient: That means that no one could ever do anything to please me. I've screamed at my kid and my wife all of my life. I give them a hard time because I expect them to know what I think without me telling them.

Physician: Have you been abusive with them?

Patient: Oh, no. Just verbally. I wouldn't hit my wife. My kid? Well, I might make him think I was going to but I never have either. I still believe in paddling a kid's bottom when he does something wrong when he is three or four years old; I mean I've done that. But I never beat him. I would never do that. The thing that might also be helpful for you to know about my family is that my father had a mental condition before he died.

Physician: What kind of condition?

Patient: He had a nervous breakdown when I was about three years old. He tried to kill himself with carbon monoxide in the garage. That's why I try to be extra strong now. I'm the breadwinner at our house, and I need to be tough. My family cusses me out and says I give them a hard time, but when it gets down to the bottom line, I'm the one they look up to. I actually function fine except I'm never happy. All I do is work. I'm forty-five years old this month, and I've never been able to do anything but work. I started working half a day when I was in grade school, so my family could eat. The times were never easy, but I always found work. I just made up my mind. That was what I had to do.

Physician: So, are you still jealous?

Patient: Am I still jealous? I guess I still wonder a little bit. I was feeling pretty bad. I am the kind of guy that if I've got a problem, I keep it to myself. If I hurt inside, I hurt and no one else knows it, if I can keep it from them.

Physician: Have you ever been unfaithful to your wife?

Patient: Maybe I have been unfaithful just once, but it was only a kiss and nothing else. A lady who painted our barn came on to me once, because like I told you, I am pretty particular in everything that I do. That means we get it right or we don't do it. She didn't do the painting to suit me, and I started getting on her case pretty heavy. I think she thought she was in trouble, so then she started being super nice to me. One day we were in a secluded place in the barn, and she came by and grabbed me, said she has had the hots for me for years, and then planted a big kiss on my lips. Things got a little out of hand there for about sixty seconds or so, and it sure never happened again. She finished the painting, and it was over. If you want to know the truth, I wish to hell it never happened.

Physician: So, do you love your wife?

Patient: Sure I love her. She is a very good lady. She works hard. We have lived together for so long we have to care a little bit for each other. But what I am trying to get across to you is that I have this coating on the outside but I have felt so bad on the inside lately. I think the only thing the antidepressant medicine did for me was make me better at hiding the hurt and anger inside.

Physician: What have you been feeling bad inside about?

Patient: I don't think my family cares for me. They tell me they do, but I don't believe it. Actions speak louder than words. I don't think my wife really cares whether I get better or not. My boy is sixteen, and when I get on him about things that he does wrong, he goes to his mother and they have a little discussion and she says: "Oh, don't pay no attention to your father."

Physician: Do you believe that?

Patient: Yes, I believe it. She says that is not so, but I see it. I may not be the smartest guy in the world, but I can find my way home. I see that. She never believed in using the paddle. According to her ways, if a kid goes into the house and picks up a bottle of something and slings it all over the walls, you're supposed to say, "Oh, you shouldn't have done that." Well, I didn't grow up that way. You whip their butt a time or two and then the next time they know better.

Physician: Is that what your dad did?

Patient: That is *exactly* what my dad did. That is what my granddad did too.

Physician: He beat you?

Patient: They both whipped me. I wouldn't say they beat me hard though. My granddad whipped my dad too.

Physician: How old were you when they whipped you?

Patient: Until I was eleven or twelve. It didn't take many whippings though. I learned real quick. Both Dad and Granddad just whipped me if I did something wrong. I wouldn't whip my son though, even if he never learns a damn thing from anybody because he's too busy talking all the time. He is at that stage where he thinks he knows everything.

Physician: Do you ever think about killing yourself?

Patient: I don't feel like I want to go out there and take a gun and blow my head off, because I know the good Lord wouldn't like it. I believe in the good Lord even though I don't go to church every Sunday. But I sure am ready to die if He is ready to take me. I work real hard, but now I just feel tired all the time. I'm just ready.

Physician: The question that I asked you is 'Are you contemplating suicide?'

Patient: No. I've told people I wish I could die, but I'm not going to shoot myself. Now what I might do is, I might get a divorce, I might just disappear, I might go somewhere and be by myself and do my own thing and say to hell with everything else.

Physician: What are you hoping that I can do for you?

Patient: I don't think there is very much that you can really do for me because I have to do it. But I think you have the training and the knowledge to get me started on the right path so I can think about the right things. I'm real good at doing stuff with my hands. If I can see someone do something once, I can do it too. More often than not, I can do it better than he can. But I've got a problem here because I can't put my hands on the part of me that's broken. I don't want to be this way.

I want to be happy and easy to get along with. I want my family to want to be around me. Now I feel like I'm going to cry. Tears seem to want to run out of my eyes every once in awhile. I'm telling you, on the outside I'm hard as rock but not on the inside.

Physician: If I am going to be your doctor, I would expect you to follow various strategies I recommend. I believe that when someone gets to the stage that you are at, you have to address the inner malady as well as maybe medicate some of the external symptoms. The way that I can help you to address the inner illness is through the use of meditation, prayer, exercise, nutrition, love, forgiveness, and ethics. These aspects are necessary to get down deep to the source of your depression.

So if we work together, it's got to be a partnership. Your end of the partnership would be to make certain promises and follow your commitments. The commitments would never go against your moral grain. I would never ask you to do anything that would offend your honor or your soul. Also, none of these steps have any negative side effects. I might say to you, "I want you to promise to exercise regularly." Or I may ask you to promise to love someone unconditionally and I would just insist that you do it.

Patient: What do you mean by love someone unconditionally? Just accept everything they do as being all right?

Physician: I am not talking about loving *what* they do. I am talking about loving that person *no matter* what they do.

Patient: I think I can do that. I am not happy with a lot of behaviors in my house, but I still stay there and make a good living for everyone. And I guarantee that if they were ever in need, I would be the first one there.

Physician: Well, making a living and taking care of a person are not necessarily the same as unconditionally loving them.

Patient: Well, I guess I don't understand. Maybe I don't know how to unconditionally love someone. Maybe I do need my inner works fixed.

　　　Now, like I said, I am pretty intense. So, let me ask you some questions. I don't know exactly how to say this because I've never really had a conversation with a doctor like this. So I will just blurt it out and maybe you can pick up bits and pieces of it: Where did you get your training that you are so much different from other doctors?

Physician: That's a great question. I've been in medical practice for thirty years. But only in the last fifteen years have I come to realize a deeper meaning to the word *practice*. What I mean is that as a physician I have learned to practice seeing my patients as spirit as much as I see them as body and mind. I have learned to practice seeing the presence of God in every one of my patients.

Patient: Let me interrupt you right there. Fifteen years ago or whenever it was, you changed your thoughts and your practice and you started down this path. You must know God pretty well.

Physician: I feel like I know to look for a Higher Power in many more places. I see God in every living thing. I see God everywhere.

Patient: You see God in every living thing? You know, I've never said this to anyone, but let me say this to you, and I can't help the tears now. They're just tears. Don't worry about them. I believe that there is nothing too big and nothing too tough to be accomplished if you have got God on your side.

Physician: I also believe that you have a healing force in you that is equivalent to the presence of God in each of your cells. Many people block their natural healing force by worry, jealousy, refusing to exercise, putting a lot of junk food in their body, and getting stressed out. My role as a physician is helping patients to get their inner-healing system working well again. I am interested in Soulful Medicine, medicine with a soul. I can teach you how to meditate to help you touch your soul. If what I am saying has some meaning to you, then we can proceed.

Patient: You think a lot the way I think about God. But the rest of what you are saying is pretty foreign to me. I don't have any idea about what you are saying to me about meditation. I understand about exercise. I can even understand the need for a good diet. But meditation, I just don't understand.

Physician: Meditation just means keeping your thoughts still—probably like being out on a starry summer night just gazing at the heavens, with nothing on your mind but the beauty of the sky. Quieting your thoughts and dwelling on peace will help stimulate your body's healing system and the production of healing chemicals called endorphins. Meditation is contemplation, a few moments to do nothing more than contemplate the presence of a Higher Power within you. It can help you find a way out of your depression.

Patient: This may be off the topic, but why do I ache so severely in my fingers and knees and back all the time when the doctors can't ever find anything wrong with me?

Physician: I can tell you for sure only after I examine you myself. However, if I found no physical abnormality, I might conclude that you ache because your physical body is just an expression of your wounded soul, a soul in turmoil. I see you as a soul afflicted with jealousy of your wife and imprinted with the memory of the violence of your upbringing. Perhaps in ways that we can't possibly understand, your feelings of depression are like your soul calling out for you to address these issues. Perhaps it is your soul seeking out care.

Patient: That's funny. The thought just went through my mind: "Wonder what brought me and this guy together." I think there is something greater than us that makes good things happen. I have never had a doctor talk to me about God. I have never, in all my life heard a doctor one time even say "Well, God bless you." I am getting this feeling that when I need help, I'm not going to be asking you, I am going to be looking inside and asking God.

Physician: That's a lovely way to put it.

Patient: Is that where I have been screwing up all this time? Is it because I don't know how to talk to God? I'm tough on the outside, but I'd get down on my knees and bawl just like a child because no matter how big you are, I believe God can hear you then.

Physician: I believe that if you just cry one tear, God will wipe away a million. So why don't you come back in a few days after you mull this over and then you can start the Wellness Rx, if that is what you want to do.

Patient: Give me a little outline here of where we start and what we'll be doing. And then tell me if it is going to cost me the farm.

Physician: It's going to cost a whole lot less than you think because I'm not going to get into a whole psychoanalysis of you here. Our work together will be very short-lived. You just have to agree to sign the Wellness Rx. Assuming personal responsibility for your own health destiny will build your self-esteem and help you to develop reverence for life. I am just going to help you to help yourself with the Wellness Rx.

Patient: I'm tough, but I am ready for help. Teach me what to do to make inside changes, because I've tried on my own. Can I start meditating even before I come back for the Wellness Rx? Can I just listen to your meditation tapes and meditate as many times as I see fit?

Physician: Listen to my tapes or use the meditation process that I will teach you as often as you want, but at least once a day until I see you again. Try to understand that your soul is in turmoil and the best way to approach the pain is to just bathe the darkness of your soul with light. Meditation will help shine that light.

Patient: So instead of jumping on my boy for not feeding the horses, I just meditate? My whole business might go right to hell.

Physician: You know what hell is? Hell is just the absence of God in your life. So if you want to get out of your hell, just invite God in. Meditation provides that invitation.

Patient: That certainly is not the version of hell I've heard about.

Physician: Hell is just the absence of a Higher Power in your life. So, let me go over a simple meditation with you now. It is just a process of quieting your thoughts and inviting in the presence of God.

Meditation Technique Practicing
the Presence of Peace

- Close your eyes and consciously relax your breathing. Breathe naturally, through your nose, and with each breath draw in a feeling of peace and calm.

- Now, take a long, even, relaxed breath, and as you exhale relax your forehead and the muscles behind your eyes.
- Take a long, even, relaxed breath, and as you exhale release the tension around your mouth, jaw, and neck.
- Take a long, even, relaxed breath, and as you exhale relax your shoulders, arms, hands, and fingers.
- Take a long, even, relaxed breath, and as you exhale let go of the tension in your chest and abdomen.
- Take a long, even, relaxed breath, and as you exhale relax the muscles throughout your back and buttocks.
- Take a long, even, relaxed breath, and as you exhale release the tension in your thighs, calves, feet, and toes.
- Take a long, even, relaxed breath, and as you exhale picture a radiant golden healing light filling your entire body from your toes to the very tip of your head.
- Continue to breathe slowly and deeply and inwardly affirm over and over to yourself: I am loved . . . I am loved . . . I am loved . . . I am loved . . . I am loved.
- Continue repeating this for as long as you wish. Before finishing, sit quietly for a moment, eyes closed, feeling the presence of peace permeating every cell of your body.

Patient: I feel relaxed, like I am floating. Like a weight has been lifted from my chest.

Physician: Yes, it's a very different feeling from just being sleepy, right? You are relaxed but you have also recharged your energy. Your endorphins are flowing, and your soul has been bathed in a healing light. The fullness of your depression makes you vulnerable, or susceptible, to real healing. When you feel darkness the most, you are closest to the light.

You are reaching out like a drowning person trying to cross a raging river of despair. I want you to know you can trust me if you reach out to me. I won't let you down. However, you must first decide whether you want to reach out. It is very important that the decision be just yours.

Patient: I am willing to reach out. But how can I get to where I'm going, to the other side of this river more quickly, and once I get there how will I stay there?

Physician: It is not like this is the rescue plan and then you are going to plunge right into it and swim ten times harder to make it work ten times faster. It doesn't work like that. It is important for you to understand that healing is a process, not an event.

Patient: But do I have to go through this continuously from now on to maintain a life without depression? How do I console myself? Is there a future down the road so a guy automatically doctors himself and doesn't realize he is doing it?

Physician: Sure. It all has to do with the unfolding and blossoming of your soul. Perhaps your soul will be expressing itself in a purer fashion than ever before, and once it has expressed itself perhaps you won't have to work so hard any more.

Patient: Is there a benefit in reading the Bible and going to church?

Physician: Absolutely. Just remember that God forgives you and that God loves you.

Patient: Sometimes I wonder if some of my depression is maybe just because I'm not as straight with God as I think I am.

Physician: And maybe some of your depression also reflects the fact that there are different passages in life like a caterpillar going into a cocoon and then emerging as a beautiful butterfly. Maybe you are in a cocoon right now, and when you come out you can be a loving and sweet individual. Maybe the pain you are experiencing is just part of shucking off that cocoon so that you can emerge as a butterfly. Once you have experienced being a butterfly you never have to go back to being a caterpillar. Come back next week for the Wellness Rx.

THE SECOND MEETING: PROMISES

Patient: The meditation relaxes me. It relaxes me so much that I can do the meditating with or without your meditation tapes.

Physician: Good. What kind of feelings does your meditating generate?

Patient: I experience a silent time. Also, I can feel the aches and pains going out of my joints when I'm meditating. I'm doing it three or four times a day.

Physician: That is a lot.

Patient: Well, I'm nervous inside, and the meditation seemed kind of like medicine. I take it and it settles me down inside.

Physician: In a sense, it is medicine, a healthy dose of peace and calm. How are you doing with your jealousy and anger?

Patient: I really haven't felt any.

Physician: Is that unusual for you?

Patient: I'll say! I have never been able to not have anger. But since the day I was here, I listen to the meditation tape in the morning, and then I just meditate out in the fields in the afternoon, and then an hour before I go to bed I do it again, and then if I wake up.

Physician: What is your usual work schedule?

Patient: Usually at eleven at night I am still in the barn shoveling hay to feed the horses. The rest of the time I'm grooming their hair, shoeing them, or washing them.

Physician: So what kind of time do you devote to your family?

Patient: I see them when they come out to the stables with me.

Physician: What type of *quality* time do you take with your wife?

Patient: Well, I'd say none. We go visit other people sometimes but rarely. We do *not* go shopping together because I hate to shop. My version of shopping is that "I need a new shovel. I know the store where I'm going to buy it. I get into the car and I drive directly there. Whatever it costs, I'll pay. I come home. It's over. I don't go to ten different stores."

Physician: Has there ever been a time when you would just take some time to sit down and chat with her?

Patient: Not really. I'm always too busy working I guess. Maybe once every four or five months we will get into the car on a Sunday afternoon and drive somewhere and eat lunch. That is about it. She is an extremely good cook, and I like to eat at home. Our quality time used to be when she and I went to bed. But now it's close to midnight, and we are usually both so tired that after fifteen minutes we are both asleep.

Physician: What is your usual pattern of sexual relations?

Patient: That sure has changed drastically. At most maybe once a week. But I'm not much interested anymore.

Physician: You may not always be an easy person to live with.

Patient: If you want to know the truth, my son tells his friends that I'm a jerk. He thinks he can't please me because I want it done so damn right that no one except God could please me. But I also know that the reason we are okay financially is because I have been particular. The question in my mind now is "Is it worth what I gave up?"

Physician: Let's talk about what you're willing to do to get your energy and happiness back. The Wellness Rx is going to require some promises on your part. The first thing I want you to promise to do is to take a brisk walk each day so that you are huffy and puffy for at least twenty minutes. While you are walking, just contemplate nature.

Patient: I'm pretty physical. I can walk home from your office if I wanted to. I live seventeen miles, but walking home wouldn't bother me at all.

Physician: Seventeen miles! You're what I would call a Type A personality. I ask you to meditate and you do it for three hours. I ask you to walk and now you want to walk seventeen miles!

Patient: I want to get well. The quicker, the better. I told you I like to see results. Any lack of results here is not going to be because I don't do what you tell me.

Physician: OK. Well, seventeen miles may be too long a walk because I know you do a lot of physical labor too. Now the next promise is to meditate every day—just like you have already been doing. Use my special meditation tape or do it by yourself.

Patient: Is there a limit to how many times a day I meditate?

Physician: No. But not all the time. I don't want you to get too wise.

Patient: I know you were kidding about meditation, but you can never know enough about anything. If I get nervous, I just like to listen to the meditation tape and it helps calm me down. So I don't think it's possible to get too wise.

Physician: You are right. OK, I see from your medical chart that you don't smoke or drink much in the way of alcohol, coffee, or soft drinks, so we don't have to spend much time on the promise that deals with addictions. So let's talk about nutrition. It is very important for you to eat high-energy, low-fat foods. Fresh fruit is available everywhere right now. I would like you to find as much fresh fruit as you can—locally grown is best because it has lots of energy. I want you to have mostly fruit until noontime because it is summer and fruit is so plentiful and good for your energy. You can have as much fruit as you wish. You can have all the apples, pears, peaches, melons, bananas—all that you want. It may make you a little gassy for a few days, but it will be all right. Eat loads and loads of fruits but not much else until noon except maybe a bowl of oatmeal and some whole-wheat bread or a bagel without butter. Can you handle that?

Patient: I promise. Cantaloupe, here I come. What do I eat the rest of the day?

Physician: It will probably require a little shift in your wife's cooking habits, but you say she is an excellent cook and I'm sure she will enjoy the recipes I am going to give you. Basically I want you to eat more vegetables, pasta, rice, baked and mashed potatoes, and whole-grain breads and cereals. Complex carbohydrates are loaded with energy.

Patient: Great. I eat loads of bread and potatoes now.

Physician: OK. But for the next seven days, do not eat any beef or pork. You can have chicken or fish on occasion, but no red meat.

Patient: Can I ask why?

Physician: The depression you are experiencing is basically a total lack of energy. It's as if your energy well has gone dry. Beef and pork take tremendous amounts of energy to digest, process, and eliminate. In exchange, they give you very little energy. And if you are out of energy, how are you going to digest the food? The purpose of the Wellness Rx is to increase your energy. The foods you will be eating are high in energy and don't require much energy to digest. That way you will have more available energy to defeat this depression. That is not to say that you can't have some beef and pork later on, but for now, live without it. If you like whole-grain cereal you can have breakfast food for lunch or dinner too. Do you drink a lot of milk or eat a lot of dairy?

Patient: Not a lot of milk, only in my cereal.

Physician: Good. You need to build up your energy, and dairy can drain your supply. By boosting your energy supply, you can help melt away your depression. You have been depressed for so long that it is affecting you at all levels—psychological, spiritual, and physical. Your depression is now as much a physical illness as a cold or a pneumonia.

Patient: I didn't realize that.

Physician: That is why antidepressant medicine is sometimes necessary. The depression has a life of its own, and you were vulnerable just like some people are vulnerable to a pneumonia when they get themselves drenched or chilled. The reason you were vulnerable is the way you were raised and the way you have led your life. Your life is apparently no longer suitable for you. You are not getting the rewards you expected from all your hard work, and you are estranged from your wife and your son. When you are doing everything you know how to do and what you know how to do is no longer suitable, that is when you become vulnerable to a bout of depression.

Now the next promise that you need to make is to live by the Golden Rule. Do you know what the Golden Rule is all about?

Patient: I can't tell you the exact words, but it is treating other people the way I want to be treated. I already try to live that way all the time. But I'm not so successful at it, either.

Physician: Here's a strategy for success. During the next week, just promise that you are not going to do anything wrong. That means don't do anything that you even *think* might be wrong. Just promise to be a kind, decent, honest, ethical, loving human being.

Patient: So if my wife wrecks the car, I need to treat her like I would want to be treated if I wrecked the car? Is that what you are saying?

Physician: Do the very, very best that you can do. Just promise to follow the Golden Rule and do nothing that you think is wrong.

Patient: Can we talk about the Golden Rule some more? If I see something that my boy needs to do, as long as I ask him to do it in a way that I would be satisfied with, I'm not supposed to yell at him? My father sure yelled at me!

Physician: Just treat your son like you would like to be treated and remember how you felt when you were being yelled at while you were growing up.

Patient: Let me say this to you. I honestly feel that a child, if you give them a few chances to do it right and you correct them very mildly and they still don't get it, I really believe that the right way is to strap them. But my son is already sixteen years old and I have sure never strapped him, so I'm just wondering.

Physician: How about just treating him with love?

Patient: I know that it is going to be tough. I love the kid inside and out. But you know, people can do some things that are against your grain so much that you just grow to despise them. My dad was the same way. So was my granddad. But if I promise, then I will just follow the Golden Rule.

Physician: That will make your next promise even easier to follow, because your next promise is to love someone unconditionally. What I mean is that no matter what the person does, you love the person, unconditionally. So, whatever it takes, hugs, kisses, smiles, quality time, a gift, anything, I am asking you for a promise of unconditional love of someone. I think it should be either your wife or your son, or even both.

Patient: The toughest one is my boy. I could love my wife very easily. But my boy would be completely different for me. If I hugged him, the kid would think I've gone off the deep end. Would it be better for my own good if I just picked my wife, because it would be a little easier to love her unconditionally for a week, or should I take on the biggest challenge in the world and choose my son? Doctor, I'll choose my wife!

Physician: The seventh and final promise may also be a challenge for you. The seventh promise I am asking you to make is to choose to be happy instead of right. In other words, all the arguments and feuds you have going on and all the lessons you are struggling to teach other people have to be suspended for seven days. That is the only way that you can be happy instead of just right.

Patient: But I have some important judgments on things. Just don't express them, is that what you are saying?

Physician: I am saying just be happy instead of insisting on being right. This will probably mean lowering some of your expectations of others for a week. Be happy, not right. You know the saying: "Judge not lest ye be judged."

Patient: OK, I agree. Maybe if I'm lucky I can get one of those sweet times when I can be both happy *and* right.

Can we go back to talking about the unconditional love promise for a moment? I just got to thinking that my son is going to leave the day after tomorrow and he will be gone the rest of the week visiting his Grandma. So it would be easy to love him too since he mostly won't be around. I mean we are talking about the next seven days, right? So I have no problem taking on the big challenge now. I will unconditionally love both my wife *and* my son.

Physician: Great. Now that doesn't mean that you go up to them and say "I'm going to love you unconditionally." Maybe just say something like this to your son: "I know I have been tough, but that is just the way that I am and it doesn't mean that I don't love you a lot, son."

Patient: That is one thing I have to admit. I'm *very* uncomfortable telling him that I love him. Even though I know it would mean a lot for both of us. I do love the boy, but I don't really know how to tell him. I'll try. That is all I can do is just try. I'm telling you though, I will have to turn around and walk off because I'll be crying.

Physician: That is all right. You don't have to worry about what you say afterward because those words will be etched in his mind forever.

Patient: I do love him, but I have done a very bad job showing it. You know if tears come to my eyes, then everybody is going to say, "Well, what is wrong with Dad? He has been the big tough guy here; what is he doing crying all of a sudden?"

Physician: How about doing something special for your wife while you are loving her unconditionally this week? Do you ever give her a gift or something?

Patient: I send her flowers once in awhile.

Physician: When was the last time you sent her flowers?

Patient: Probably five years ago.

Physician: Would you do that again?

Patient: Yes.

Physician: Please sign the Wellness Rx now, and I'll see you in seven days.

OUR NEXT VISIT: A LIGHT FROM WITHIN

Patient: I have been on the Wellness Rx for a whole week now. I honestly think I am doing great. From where I sit and from what I know, the world is treating me good. I feel a lot better inside.

Physician: You feel better inside. What does that mean?

Patient: I'm not down. Don't get me wrong, I have moments. It seems like a light switch goes off at times and then I feel depressed again. But most of the time I feel a lot better. I feel so much better inside. I don't think I realized how low I was.

I have a totally different outlook on my son. It's like a miracle. He was really my problem because I couldn't communicate with him. I couldn't get him to listen to the things that I wanted him to know and the louder I talked the farther we grew apart. To be honest with you, it was so bad that I actually sort of despised him. Now I don't feel that way.

I promised to love my son unconditionally, and I'll be the first to tell you that I didn't do very good at all the first day. He and I got into it. We had it up one side and down the other just like always. But later on that day I just took him by the shoulders and told him that I loved him. I said I didn't mean the stuff I said to him, and it seems that we have a wonderful relationship right now. I want my son to turn out real good, and I want him to have respect for me. I think I was getting close to the point of losing him completely. But now I have hope for the first time that we will become closer. Maybe a little bit of me is showing him how much I really care for him. Does this mean anything to you?

Physician: It is more important that it means something to you. The Wellness Rx is designed to work quickly. It's like throwing a life preserver to a person in need. How about the rest of your promises?

Patient: I am meditating every day. I think I am becoming an expert at it. I have also been exercising a lot. I start to walk for twenty minutes and it ends up being about three miles. I walk pretty fast too.

Physician: What about nutrition? Are you eating lots of fruits, vegetables, and complex carbohydrates—rice, pasta, potatoes, whole-grain breads?

Patient: You bet, and I have had no red meat and just two pieces of chicken all week.

Physician: How are you doing with loving your wife unconditionally?

Patient: It is so easy.

Physician: Why?

Patient: Because for the first time I am really practicing seeing God in every living thing, especially in my wife. I don't know how I could have missed this before.

Physician: Perhaps you missed it because of the way you had been taught to think when you were a little boy. How young were you when you first learned to think that a wife is not an equal?

Patient: I was probably four or five years old. I grew up in a house and a family where the woman was supposed to be a half-step behind.

Physician: What did you learn about what men were supposed to do in the home you grew up in?

Patient: I grew up learning that I was supposed to be strong and macho. Dad just got up in the morning and left for work each day, trying to be the breadwinner. Until he had a nervous breakdown and tried to kill himself. Mom stayed home and did the housework, and Dad made all the decisions.

Physician: So, in a way, you learned that women are kind of inferior to men. Treat them better than the horses, but not like trusted, loving friends.

Patient: Exactly. And sometimes in my case, I've not even treated them as well as the horses. But to be honest with you, I am ready to turn my back on those ways. You are breaking new ground for me and I am learning and hopefully taking it all in and expanding my horizons.

Physician: I think that you are too, because once you become aware of this, all you *can* do is expand. However, since your past is still a part of you, you can't just cut it out. But what you can do is turn to the light. Shine the light in that darkness in your soul. We talked initially about how your depression is a reflection of your soul in turmoil. Now you can light it up. That is what we are trying to do together. Directing you toward the light of your soul.

Patient: I understand that very plainly.

Physician: Good, then I want you to sign here that you will continue following the Wellness Rx for another week.

Patient: Gladly. We are on the track now. When we first started talking I was locked into thinking down a track that was wrong. Sometimes though, you are coming at me with so much new stuff that I can't figure it all out. You know why I try to figure everything out? I want to make sure nobody is taking me down a deep, dark path and getting me lost.

Physician: The only thing that you have to figure out is how far the concept of a Higher Power being everywhere and in every living thing can take you. Also, the reason you try to figure everything out is because you have been taught to be suspicious. Now the ways that you have been taught to think have stopped working for you. Instead of getting to the other side of the river called "middle age," you began drowning. You have broken free of the current now, and you are almost over to the other side. The Wellness Rx is your life preserver. You can get safely to the other side by taking personal responsibility for your health destiny and developing self-esteem and reverence for life. So keep all your promises and I will see you next week. If you are willing to say yes to God by doing all this, then God is going to say yes, yes, yes to you. *That's the way it all works.*

Patient: Maybe this is not the place to say this, but each time I come to see you I develop more faith in you. I think you have done a real good job so far, and you are teaching me some very valuable things about life.

Physician: Thank you. And you are teaching me too.

OUR FINAL VISIT: LOOKING BACKWARD, LIVING FORWARD

Life can only be understood backwards; it has to be lived forwards.
—*Søren Kierkegaard*

Physician: Boy, do you look good!

Patient: Thank you. Thank you.

Physician: I mean, you look *really* good!

Patient: Well, I have been feeling pretty decent.

Physician: What is happening? You look about seven years younger.

Patient: I have to say that looking in the mirror I thought I looked pretty good this morning too. It seemed like I had more pink in my face. As far as I know, everything is going fine.

Physician: Let's go over our contract now. How are you doing with the nutrition?

Patient: Just fine.

Physician: So, are you eating fruits, vegetables, and complex carbohydrates—all the food that's full of life and energy?

Patient: Loads of it, and the only flesh I've had this week is some fish, just once. I have fresh-squeezed orange juice in the morning and then cantaloupe, a banana, or maybe some pears. In the afternoon, I eat a sandwich with lettuce and sliced tomatoes on some whole-wheat or pita bread. My wife uses the recipe for the terrific honey mustard dressing your nurse gave her. For dinner I have mashed or baked potatoes and more vegetables or pasta or something like that. I thought it would be hard not to eat beef because we have been meat-and-potato eaters for years. But I feel so much better now that it is not worth going back to beef and pork again. Actually, I think I'd gag.

Physician: Good. There is a little bit of the vegetarian in everyone. The point of this whole nutrition plan is to build up your energy to help your own healing forces get to work.

Patient: Speaking of energy, I am walking real rapidly through the woods now about a mile every morning and night. I'm really enjoying meditating. I meditate at least once a day. I go into the bedroom and lay down on the bed and listen to your meditation tape, or I just sit under a tree, close my eyes, and do it myself.

Physician: How did you get along with your wife and son and your promises of unconditional love? And what about following the Golden Rule?

Patient: I am doing real good. I don't know, but it is just no big deal anymore. It is so much easier than it was before.

Physician: Since healing is a process, not an event, I want you to continue doing everything you are doing now. However, now I want you to love *yourself* unconditionally too. That may be a little hard because you give yourself a pretty tough time now and then.

Patient: I am pretty bad about putting myself down.

Physician: You have put yourself down for not living up to your own expectations. Maybe those expectations are unreasonable or just no longer work for you. I would like to point out to you that by signing the Wellness Rx and living up to your commitments, you are taking a major step toward defining a new you.

You are establishing an entirely new ethic, laying down new mental blueprints. You are defining who you really are. You make a commitment and then you live up to the commitment. Then your commitment achieves definition, solidity, and reality. In a sense, it is almost like creating spiritual alchemy. You are becoming a spiritual individual, dedicated to integrity, which means living up to your promises.

Finally, it is never too late to have a happy childhood, and that is what you are now creating for yourself. The negative memories of your childhood, the ones that led you toward putting down women, screaming at your son, or punishing yourself, are being neutralized. You are building new memories of good people, good incidents, and good experiences.

I want to tell you that your wife called me yesterday to tell me how wonderful she thinks you are doing, how much she loves and respects you for making these promises and fulfilling them. She wanted me to know what a difference she sees in you.

Patient: Now I know she loves me too. I want to be honest with you. I have been studying myself a lot lately. When I see something broken, I analyze it and then fix it myself. When I first came to see you, I knew there was something wrong, but I had no idea where to begin to fix it or how.

Now I realize that I have not really been living as myself, who I really am. I grew up a young child being pretty timid and shy. It was as if one day a truck dumped the old, cruel world on me. My dad got sick and I had to start working. I had to make some money, and I found out real quick that out in the real world, things aren't always fair. It seemed like overnight, I put on a big suit of armor, the shell of a tough guy. But inside, I'm not tough at all. Probably for thirty years I have lived that, and it has not been me at all. I guess I didn't know any other way. I had forgotten the tender, gentle way to live, or I guess I had never learned it. Hopefully, I can get that turned around, because something, I can't tell you what it is, but something has now drastically changed inside me.

Physician: You were drowning in a raging river of no return because all you ever learned to do was to be more tough and to work even harder. You were trying to get from one shore of your life to another, and you couldn't make it by just swimming harder. That suit of armor was weighing you down, pulling you under. No wonder you felt like you were going down. Now be true to your self. You learned a lot of lessons growing up. A lot of ways to think. But those are not your self. Your Self with the big "S" is your inner light, your soul. Spiritually and emotionally you have been shipwrecked, and you were just looking for something to hang on to when you came to see me.

Patient: Honestly, I can look in a mirror and I can tell that I have an enlightened look. And I feel better. I look doggone good, let me tell you. And mostly I feel so much better inside.

Physician: I am pleased that you have done so remarkably well. It's crucially important for you to stay with the program. Don't veer from the wellness path now. You've emerged from the dark cocoon of depression into the world of the butterfly. I think our work together is finished. God bless you.

> *The man with the clear head is the*
> *man who . . . looks life in the face,*
> *and feels himself lost . . .*
> *instinctively, as do the shipwrecked,*
> *he will look around for something*
> *to which to cling*
> *and that tragic glance, absolutely sincere,*
> *will cause him to bring order*
> *into the chaos of his life.*
>   *—José Ortega Y Gasset*

13
SAYING GOOD NIGHT TO INSOMNIA

Who looks outside, dreams.
Who looks inside, wakes.

—*C. G. Jung*

This Insomnia Wellness Rx builds upon the basic Wellness Rx outlined in Chapter Two to provide the necessary pillars of support for a good night's sleep. In addition to the seven basic promises of the Wellness Rx, the following components are geared specifically toward overcoming insomnia.

THE EIGHT COMPONENTS FOR A GOOD NIGHT'S SLEEP

If you are having trouble sleeping, add the eight components presented here to the seven promises of the Wellness Rx.

- Create a sleepy environment
- Cultivate a therapeutic sleep routine
- Put worries to rest
- Avoid uppers and downers
- Eliminate unnecessary prescription drugs
- Create a personal bedtime story
- Establish a personal code of honor
- Have mercy on yourself

Sixty years ago Dr. Walter B. Cannon introduced the word *homeostasis*, defining it as "the body at peace with itself." Homeostasis is indeed the secret to a restful night's sleep. I have previously introduced an expanded definition of *homeostasis* to include peace of mind and soul as well. I find it amazing that so many patients complain to me of problems with sleeping. Statistics actually show that one-third of Americans have difficulty sleeping, and one out of five doctor's office visits are for insomnia. About twelve million Americans, twice as many women as men, will visit their doctors this year for insomnia. Doctors will write about twenty-two million prescriptions for sleeping pills to sedate wide-awake brains without addressing the problems underlying their sleeplessness. Stress is not only disrupting health and happiness, it's interrupting our sleep.

This Insomnia Wellness Rx is designed to uproot the underlying troubles that are keeping you awake at night. It will help you alleviate your difficulties falling asleep and staying asleep by fueling homeostasis, your natural Healing Force. The first important thing to understand is that there is no "right amount" or "wrong amount" of sleep for you. Most adults will feel best when they sleep between six and eight hours each day. However, many people do well with as little as five or six hours of sleep a night, and others feel best after nine or ten hours of rest. The amount of sleep you need may even be genetically influenced and therefore similar to what your parents required.

The second important point to keep in mind is that your sleep requirement changes at various times in your life. Infants wake up frequently, and children sleep for long periods. Young adults generally sleep through the night. Then, with more age, sleep is naturally interrupted by periods of wakefulness that don't necessarily detract from a good night's sleep. Whereas most younger to middle-aged adults feel great with eight hours of sleep, six hours usually feels fine to people in their seventies.

If you think you are losing sleep by tossing and turning all night, endlessly ruminating and thinking, the third thing to know is that you may actually be sleeping a lot more than you imagine. What feels like an hour and a half of staring wide-eyed at the dark is often just fifteen minutes when measured. True insomnia means regular difficulty in falling asleep or staying asleep when your mind and body really need to be asleep. If you experience prolonged periods of restless tossing and turning while trying to sleep and are subsequently tired and irritable, this Insomnia Wellness Rx can help you get the night's rest you have been waiting for.

Many uncommon sleep disorders are currently gaining much attention in the popular press. Sleep apnea is a frequently cited yet unusual cause of sleeplessness. Affected individuals are usually obese, male, and heavy snorers. People with sleep apnea repeatedly cease to breathe while asleep and then wake up gasping for breath. This unfortunate cycle occurs throughout the night. Some sleep apnea sufferers have no memory of waking up but feel extremely groggy the next day. In my thirty years of family medicine practice I have not encountered or recognized a sleep apnea patient, but the literature suggests their numbers are increasing. (Speak with your physician if the above description appears applicable to you.)

Your Healing Force naturally directs your mind and body to a good night's rest so that you will be recharged and ready to go the next day. Sleeplessness often results from an energy imbalance. Lack of sleep may come to you if your emotional and mental tensions are running too high. Conversely, sleeplessness itself can upset your energy balance and cause mental, physical, or emotional illness. Thus, insomnia is an internally driven classic vicious circle. The more your sleep is disrupted today, the more likely it is to be disturbed tomorrow; the more stress you are feeling, the less easily sleep will come; the more poorly you sleep, the more likely your stress will multiply since your resources for distilling stress will be exhausted. Fortunately, you can intervene in this circle and stop its power to keep you awake at night.

The first step is to determine whether you really need the sleep you are not getting. Is it possible you may just need to go to sleep later or wake up earlier? Only you know the answer. If indeed you are really losing much-needed sleep and as a result feel tired and ineffective the next day, then this Insomnia Wellness Rx will help you intervene in the disruptive cycle of sleeplessness you are caught in. This prescription puts you in charge and will work only if you are willing to take personal responsibility for fulfilling each of its components. This Insomnia Wellness Rx is meaningful and clinically effective only after you sign the prescription and then follow it exactly. Only total commitment will bring results. This advice is meaningless and will not help you sleep unless you follow through with your promises.

If what you want to do is sleep, then follow the guidelines for a deep rest described in the remainder of this chapter.

CREATE A SLEEPY ENVIRONMENT

The first step toward sleep is creating an environment conducive to sleeping. A comfortable bed and clean sheets are obviously not enough if you are having trouble sleeping. You may need to go a little bit overboard, but surely it will be worth it if you can return to regular, peaceful sleeping patterns.

- *Sound.* Studies tracking the brain-wave patterns of people at sleep indicate that noise lessens the depth of sleep. Even if you *think* that you are used to the noise in your environment, it may be keeping you from deep sleep. Do what you can to shut out noise in your bedroom. For noise you can't control, such as traffic or the neighbor's automatic sprinkler system, soft, moldable ear plugs can be very helpful. Many people find that using only one ear plug in the ear not pressed against the pillow is sufficient.

- *Ventilation, temperature, and humidity.* An open window, even in cold weather, can often encourage sleep. It doesn't have to be the window directly over your bed and may even be the window in your bathroom. Throw on an extra blanket, use a down comforter, or even some flannel sheets. With a warm covering the fresh, cool night air won't give you a cold, but it will enhance your sleep. Sometimes just a change in your sleeping environment will solve your sleeplessness. Try pajamas if you sleep naked, or try sleeping naked if you wear pajamas. Control the humidity if the heater is on, because it dries your sinuses and nasal passages. A dry throat or nose will cause you to wake. Get a humidifier or put some bowls of water in the corners of your bedroom if you are unable to control the heater.

- *Night light.* Some people sleep best in pitch dark, while others are more comfortable with a sliver of light coming from beneath a closed door. If you are trying unsuccessfully to fall asleep in absolute darkness, turn on a light in the hallway or bathroom and leave your door open a crack. If you normally try to sleep with a bit of light but are not falling asleep, turn the light off.

- *Mattress and pillow comfort.* A firm or soft pillow or mattress is a matter of personal preference. Some people like two pillows, and others just one. Again, if whatever you are using is not entirely comfortable, then a change is in order. Also, if your bedmate reminds you of a lumbering dinosaur, you might consider a king-sized mattress or separate single ones, side by side.

Therapeutic Sleep Routine

For many people suffering from insomnia, even the sight of their bed makes them anxious about falling asleep. That anxiety itself—the simple thought, "I wonder if I'll fall asleep easily tonight"—can cause sleeplessness. The following steps will help you uproot those negative mental blueprints and cultivate a mental association between your bedroom and easy sleep.

- *Use your bedroom only for sleeping, meditation, nighttime reading, and sex.* This will help you associate your bedroom with relaxing and sleepiness. Don't use it for daytime reading, telephoning, watching television, eating, studying, working, or finishing "projects."
- *Get out of bed at roughly the same time each day,* even if you had trouble sleeping the night before. Don't get into the habit of sleeping later to make up for lost sleep the night before. This may make you feel better temporarily, but when it comes to sleeping the next night you will most likely find it even harder to fall asleep.
- *Go to bed only when you really feel sleepy.*
- *Meditate in bed just before you go to sleep.*
- *Avoid naps.* If you must doze off, limit your nap to under an hour and take it before two in the afternoon.
- *Take a long, hot bath or shower before bedtime.* The warm water relaxes your muscles and soothes your body. Take extra time for yourself to leisurely brush and floss your teeth and enjoy giving yourself a facial or even shave for the next day.
- *Restrict what you drink* in the hour or two before your bedtime to what you need to rinse after brushing and to swallow any medications. Avoid drinking much during the night, since lying down seems to stimulate the need to urinate, a sensation that increases with age.
- *Read a magazine or good book once you are under the covers.* Definitely stay away from "spine tinglers" or "can't-put-it-down" books, since these will stimulate rather than relax and calm you. Try something uplifting, amusing, biographical, informative, or inspirational—anything that encourages a quiet mind and rest.
- *A cup of decaffeinated herbal tea,* perhaps with a bit of honey, at bedtime is soothing. Chamomile tea is especially comforting. Valerian root, available in capsules or as a tea, is an herbal preparation I recommend to patients and is available from health-food stores. Although it encourages sleep, it does not smell so good, however. Read the label on your tea carefully to be sure it does not contain caffeine, and don't drink a tea that is especially spicy, since this will stimulate your senses rather than calm you for sleep.

- *If there is a television in your bedroom, consider moving it to another room.* Watch your television news in the morning or early evening but never before you go to bed. The news can be upsetting and disturbing, and the violent or sad images you see may stay in your mind as you try to sleep. If you are addicted to nighttime talk shows, just shut the TV off. Tape the show with a video recorder and watch it in the morning as you get ready for work.

- *Sex is usually helpful.* If you are having a disagreement with your bed partner, be sure to resolve it before you get into bed. Never go to sleep angry. Remember your promise to "be happy, not right," which you may also take to mean in this instance: "be sleepy, not right."

- *If you are experiencing physical pain, don't try to "tough it out."* Take 400 mg ibuprofen, two aspirin, or two acetaminophen tablets before you go to sleep, especially if you are suffering from muscle, joint, or headache pain.

- *Lying in bed wide awake for too long will only make matters worse.* If you can't get to sleep and you've been tossing and turning for what seems like much too long, then get up and do something else. Put on the light and read in bed. If you sleep beside someone, buy a small reading light so that you don't keep him or her awake. Or put on something comfortable and go into another room. Relax and watch television (remember, no news), listen to music, pay bills, catch up on correspondence, do filing, do the wash, or finish some chores. Don't give in to frustration. Being frustrated over not sleeping only fuels your sleeplessness. A poor night of sleep every once in a while is absolutely not going to hurt you. It is usually not even necessary to make up for it the next night. Make lemonade out of a midnight lemon by just enjoying some extra quiet time or accomplishing something unexpected.

- *Get lots of daylight, sunshine, and fresh air.* Make every attempt to fulfill your promise to exercise by doing it outdoors. Exercise in the afternoon or the very early evening for a good night's sleep, but not within two hours of bedtime.

- *Eat very little after dinner and limit any snacking to a piece of fresh fruit.* A banana or an apple will satisfy you and have a calming effect. Absolutely do not eat any sweets. Remember that food is energy, and different kinds of foods affect your energy in different ways. When the energy of refined sugar hits your brain it generates endless thoughts that roll around in your head and make you roll around restlessly in your bed. Avoid high fat at dinner. Beef, pork, gravy, butter, and ice cream require enormous amounts of energy to digest. All that activity in your stomach and intestines can contribute to your restlessness. It is hard for your body to relax and your mind to quiet down when your stomach and intestines are working overtime. The best evening meal for a good night's sleep consists of complex carbohydrates, whole grains, and vegetables. Pasta with tomato sauce and some salad or a hearty vegetable soup with some fresh bread will have a calming effect and won't keep your stomach busy through the night.

PUT WORRIES TO REST

Ask people who have ever had difficulty sleeping what keeps them awake at night, and they will usually tell you it is worry. People who have problems falling to sleep are typically people with a lot of worries on their mind. When the worrier hits the pillow, his or her mind goes into overdrive. If you spend the moments (or hours) before you drift off to sleep worrying about things, there are three things to remember about worry that will help you put your worries to rest so that you can get some sleep.

- *Worry is never of benefit.* Keep a notepad or index cards with a pencil or pen at your bedside. Keep in mind that 95 percent of what you worry about will never happen and the rest you have little or no control over. If you start to worry about forgetting something that you think you should remember, then just write it down so you won't worry about forgetting it anymore.

   Worry feeds on itself and multiplies in your mind. Worry makes you forget that your worry is just your very own thoughts doing the worrying. Your own thoughts begin thinking that what you are worrying about is *real* instead of merely what you are thinking. So if you are worried about forgetting something, you can immediately ease your mind by writing it down instead of tossing and turning in bed. Free your mind of worry so that you can put it to sleep.

- *Worry never helps.* If your worry has become so real to you that you surely know that you won't forget it, but nevertheless it still keeps running around in your mind, then write down that worry too. The next step is to list three actions that you can take to help eliminate the particular worry. Be brief and concise about your solutions. Do this for each worry. Pretty soon you will teach your mind that the worry is not worth the effort it takes you to switch on the light, pick up the pen, and write down your worries and steps to reduce them. Examples:

  Worry: No money for Christmas gifts.
  Action: (1) Make gift baskets of homemade cookies; (2) knit socks; (3) paint small pictures; (4) ask for salary advance.

  Worry: Mother is getting forgetful and can't see at night.
  Action: (1) Phone brother, sister, father; (2) consider moving closer; (3) suggest bus instead of driving; (4) make doctor's appointment to check for cataracts.

  Worry: Too many projects going on.
  Action: (1) Delay a project; (2) postpone a business trip; (3) get a computer.

- *Worry is entirely a product of your imagination.* Your thoughts are being generated by what you read in newspapers, magazines, and books and by what you watch and hear on television, radio, and in the movies. Your brain is mercilessly bombarded with disturbing stimuli every moment you are awake. The primary reason why you have trouble sleeping is likely to be that your mind and emotions are running so fast and receiving so much sensory information that it is impossible to process it all.

  You are either overexcited and anticipating something or are afraid and apprehensive of something. Either way, it is all in your mind. You may not be able to control people, circumstances, or events, but you can control your reactions and responses to them. You can learn to manage your worry. The crucial point that you must understand about worry management is that you cannot use your worried thoughts to solve what you are worried about. You need to clear your mind of worry before you can manage your worries. The Insomnia Wellness Rx helps you put your worries to rest.

Avoid Uppers and Downers

- *Do not drink alcohol at least eight hours before bedtime.* Alcohol is a depressant that makes you feel drowsy initially, but the older you get, the more it interferes with your sleep. After the initial drowsiness wears off, alcohol wakes you up two or three hours after you have fallen asleep. Once you are awake, the lingering effects of alcohol can encourage your thoughts to race about willy-nilly for hours on end.

- *Drink no more than one cup of caffeinated coffee in the morning.* Don't drink coffee or caffeinated tea any later in the day. Two cans of caffeinated soda is about equal to a cup of coffee. I suggest that you don't drink caffeinated sodas at all. As you age you become more sensitive to caffeine so that while it may not have been a problem before, it may very well become a problem later on. Caffeine does not belong in your daily menu if you are having a problem sleeping.

- *Nicotine is a stimulant that affects the heart, blood vessels, and nervous system as well as every cell in your body.* The more cigarettes you smoke, the more difficulty sleeping you are likely to have. While it is important to quit for your general health, if you want to sleep better, smoke less before bedtime.

- *Over-the-counter sleeping pills are not generally helpful.* They usually contain antihistamines, mainly used for congestion and allergies, which cause drowsiness. Unfortunately, they also tend to just dry out your nasal passages and may cause irritability, nervousness, and confusion. If you feel that you occasionally must have a little "something" to sleep, a useful alternative to the expensive brands with multiple chemicals is meclizine, a nonprescription medicine used to avert seasickness but which also induces sleep. Instead of a sleeping pill, take one meclizine 25 mg tablet at bedtime. Remember, this too is a drug and should not be taken on a regular basis.

Eliminate Unnecessary Prescription Drugs

Prescription sleeping pills may help you fall asleep, but they do not help you sleep "well." They do nothing to help reverse the reason for your sleeplessness in the first place. I prescribe sleeping pills on occasion, but only as a temporary solution for an acute problem or an emotional crisis. If you take sleeping pills for more than a few days, your body begins to expect the drug, and you have to pay the price of forgetfulness or a mental and physical hangover. Sleeping pills are just not helpful for regular insomnia because all they do is mask the underlying source of your sleeplessness. Moreover, if you become dependent on the sleeping pills, you begin to require larger doses that can then be dangerous, especially if you mix them with alcohol or other prescription or over-the-counter drugs. If you are already dependent on sleeping pills, be sure to withdraw from them only gradually. Cut your dose in half every three or four days. Barbiturates especially can cause dangerous problems if you stop "cold turkey."

Halcion, Dalmane, Restoril, Doral, Placidyl, phenobarbital, and the more than one hundred brands of sleeping pills available by prescription will not address the problem underlying your sleeplessness. The reason you are not sleeping is because your energy is out of balance or disturbed. The pills may just further perturb your homeostasis. There was a time when doctors would occasionally and judiciously administer a sedative for the pangs of childbirth or the immediate grief of losing a loved one. Now, however, pervasive stress combined with profit motives of drug companies causes the ludicrous drugging of tens of millions of people into an unnatural sleep each night. Senior citizens especially seem to be regarded as a natural receptacle for pills. Consider the following stunning statistics:

- Approximately 90 percent of Americans over the age of sixty take at least one prescription drug regularly, and tens of millions take two to four prescription drugs simultaneously.

- Sixty percent of Americans between the ages of sixty-five and eighty-four take at least three different prescription drugs a year; 37 percent take five prescription drugs a year; and 19 percent are taking seven or more prescription drugs each year.

- About ten million adverse drug reactions occur yearly in older Americans, and harmful reactions to drugs cause approximately 275,000 adults over the age of sixty to be hospitalized every year. As we age our bodies take more time to metabolize medicine and the doses just accumulate in the body's system.

But older Americans are not the only ones whose balance of energy is disrupted by sleeping pills. All of these drugs just compound the sleeping problem, whether you are age twenty-five or seventy-five, because they do not address the reasons for your sleeplessness in the first place. Often sleeplessness occurs as a side effect of some other prescription drug you may be taking. In fact, a random browse through the *Physician's Desk Reference*, which lists the adverse effects of every drug, reveals that an overwhelming majority of all drugs have been determined to cause insomnia. What the *PDR* does not show is the sleeplessness factor that results from combining two or more particular prescription drugs. Here is an actual list of seventeen drugs regularly taken by a sixty-eight-year-old woman who came to see me for insomnia and swollen ankles:

Atarax	Isordil	Ornade	Tolinase
Atavan	Keflex	Parafon Forte	Zantac
Catapres	Lasix	Proloprim	
Darvon	Maxzide	Synthroid	
Halcion	Mevacor	Tagamet	

For eight of the drugs listed, the *PDR* indicates insomnia as a possible adverse reaction! Unfortunately, there is no database from which it is possible to calculate what drugs can do *in combination* with each other. Insomnia is even identified as a side effect of the two sedative prescriptions that this patient was taking to sleep!

Americans are by far the most medicated people in the world, and it is important that you ask your physician whether you really need all of the medicines you are taking in the doses that you are taking them. Do *not* stop your prescription medications other than perhaps your nonbarbiturate sleeping pills without the agreement of your physician.

Night Shifts and Sunday Night Crazies

Perhaps the most frequent sufferers of insomnia are the tens of millions of Americans who work night shifts. Human body rhythms are intricately connected with the rising and setting of the sun. Attuned to these circadian rhythms, it is simply more natural for humans to rise when the sun rises and to sleep when the sun falls. If you work at night and have trouble sleeping during the day, the optimal solution, in terms of your sleep, is to switch to a daytime work schedule. Of course, this may be impractical or impossible for a number of reasons. If you cannot make the switch to a daytime job, then make an extra effort to keep your bedroom as dark and as quiet as possible when you go to bed. In a few days you can get your inner clock to behave as if you were sleeping after the sun has gone down. By all means, try to maintain a similar sleep schedule on the days that you are not working, and pay particular attention to adequate exercise and to eliminating alcohol, tobacco, and caffeine from your life. Make sure to follow all of the recommendations of the Insomnia Wellness Rx so that you can have a good day's sleep.

Weekends make us do crazy things. We tend to let loose on the weekend after working hard all week. Almost everyone it seems gets caught up in the struggle to get a good night's sleep Sunday night to be fresh and alive Monday morning. We climb into bed Sunday night and hope to make up for late weekend nights, too many drinks, too many televised football games, and too many indiscretions of all sorts that go beyond the bounds of moderation. We also tend to sleep in late on weekend mornings.

So by the time Sunday night rolls around, our inner time clocks have been thrown off balance. We lie awake staring at the ceiling, tossing and turning while waiting impatiently for sleep to come. Most people will not like the sound of the easiest solution to their Sunday night frustration: MODERATION. If you don't see yourself willing to give up late weekend nights or a few beers, perhaps you can agree to the following:

- On the weekends get out of bed at the same time you wake during the week or not more than one hour later, regardless of how late you stayed up or what you did the night before.
- Get as much fresh air and sunshine as you can during the weekends.

In any case, while you may drag around on Monday morning, an occasional poor night's sleep will never hurt you, and Monday night will feel awfully good.

Create a personal bedtime story as described in the following section, to focus your attention from elsewhere, to within. When you lie awake in bed trying to fall asleep, all of your attention is focused on your unsuccessful attempts at slumber. Your attention is fixed on the clock and how long it seems since you first slipped into bed. You put your attention into worrying that without a good night's sleep you will perform inadequately at work the next morning. Great amounts of your attention are directed at determining exactly how many hours of sleep you can still get if you fall asleep by a particular time. The attention you pay to the clock or to your failed efforts at sleep will only make things worse. Directing your attention and focus within, on your own soothing and comforting memories, will help you to shut out all of the worries, fears, anxieties, and despair that are keeping sleep at bay in the first place. Training your mind to linger quietly over a touching personal story will train your body to fall asleep easily, soundly, without struggle.

CREATE A PERSONAL BEDTIME STORY

One of the most comforting things about childhood was the stories we were told to send us off to sleep. In nearly every culture, in nearly every language, children around the world are put to sleep with a soothing story. The Insomnia Wellness Rx reinvents this tradition for adults and asks you to create your own personal bedtime story. For one week, every night, tell yourself this story as you try to doze off. The story should be warm, loving, and peaceful. It should include nature, and people you love and care for. The story should be essentially true, but use your imagination and be creative.

Maybe your story goes back to your childhood and recalls a moment when you felt especially safe and loved. Perhaps your story recalls a special occasion, a special Christmas with the entire family and a warm fireplace. Or maybe your bedtime story is based on a fond memory of your mother teaching you how to bake bread or fly a kite. Or is your story about telling your own child a bedtime story and his sleepy smile as he falls asleep? Whatever your story is about, it should call forth images of friendliness, peace, warmth, safety, comfort, calm, and love.

ESTABLISH A PERSONAL CODE OF HONORING YOURSELF

The outward purpose of your personal bedtime story is to soothe you to sleep. The inward deeper purpose of your story is to help you uncover and transform pain that you have not successfully managed to let go. Establishing a personal code of honoring yourself will help you let go of these pains and in turn will free you from the restlessness that keeps you awake nights.

Nearly each and every one of us carries buried within a handful of unspoken pains. This should come as no surprise. The world we live in offers very little relief from pain and worry. We have to seek this relief within ourselves, in the deepest part of us, our souls. The basic seven promises of the Wellness Rx help you find this inner source of peace. In addition to those basic promises, the Insomnia Wellness Rx helps you develop a personal code of honor. Honoring yourself and the goodness within you is like a cradle that will rock you gently to sleep. So for the week of your Insomnia Rx, adopt and follow this personal code: *"I will love myself no matter what I have done and no matter what I have been through."*

To ensure a long and restful night's sleep, keep this personal code of honoring your goodness in your mind and heart while you tell yourself your bedtime story. If you start to lose your concentration because other thoughts come creeping in, just refocus your attention again and again. Pay particular attention to any negative memories that interfere with your story. Simply by affirming that you love yourself no matter what you have done and no matter what you have been through, you will drive those negative memories away.

It is actually never too late to have a happy childhood. Just consider for a moment what your mind is made up of. Psychologists and philosophers have been thinking about this puzzle for centuries. Today it is generally believed that much of the work that goes on in your mind is under the command of your ego, the cerebral stuff with which your mind thinks. Your ego is formed by every experience, learning episode, adventure, and misadventure you have ever lived through. It consists of all the virtues and prohibitions you learned from those you have loved as well as from those you have feared. Basically, your ego is the conglomeration of all your thoughts, attitudes, impressions, and opinions.

In his book *Wisdom of the Ego,* George E. Valiant suggests that the two main characteristics of a healthy and mature ego are resilience and the ability to sustain paradoxes. Sustain paradoxes? Yes, to accept contradictions. It is possible, therefore, to reprogram your ego. As long as you are willing to take personal responsibility to be the very best person you can, your ego is inclined to help you love yourself no matter what you have done and for whatever you have been through. Contradiction, the poet Walt Whitman proclaimed, is inherently human: "Do I contradict myself? Very well then, I contain multitudes."

Every human being contains multitudes, multiple layers of identity and self constantly being revealed as we grow, mature, and change. The Insomnia Wellness Rx encourages your awareness of your own multitudes and helps you develop greater self-value and reverence for life. Your ego's built-in capacity to sustain paradoxes allows you to regard yourself as worthy and good no matter what you have done or what you have been through. **It is as if your mind declares a general amnesty and you are forgiven.** If your religious beliefs require redemption, repentance, and atonement, the Wellness Rx embraces that for you. If your religious beliefs require a constant turning toward God's eternal grace, the Wellness Rx embraces that for you too.

> *My religion is very simple. My religion is kindness.*
> —*The Dalai Lama*

Another important attribute of a healthy and maturing ego is a sense of spiritual awe, a sense of something beyond the ego's grasp. The poet Edward Arlington Robinson likened the world to a spiritual kindergarten, inhabited by millions of bewildered infants trying to spell God with the wrong blocks. The Insomnia Wellness Rx leads you to graduate to a new set of blocks: a series of promises you make to yourself to take personal responsibility for your health destiny. These are the building blocks to a good night's rest.

It has been said that the human mind can make a hell out of heaven or a heaven out of hell. Worry, fear, anxiety, and despair are the four walls surrounding the hellish experience of insomnia. The promises constituting the Insomnia Wellness Rx are the pathways that lead you from the dread of insomnia to sound, heavenly, peaceful slumber. As you tell yourself your bedtime story, charting your way to a peaceful night's rest, your worries and fears, including the memories of destructive relationships and shameful acts, will involuntarily come to mind and disrupt your comforting narrative. These meanderings are just a reflection of the restlessness in your soul. Know that you can redefine your past as well as rehearse a future at peace with yourself. Your bedtime story is a strategy for sublime transformation in the here and now.

Confirm your resolve to just honor your goodness and a good night's rest by signing the Insomnia Wellness Rx. Doing so will help awaken the quality of spiritual awe in your ego. Just pay attention to your personal code of honor while you are telling yourself your bedtime story: *I will love myself no matter what I have done and no matter what I have been through.*

Have Mercy on Yourself

I recently came across a tale about an encounter between a Zen master and his student that illustrates the simple lessons of this chapter. Wellness, and specifically a well night's rest, really requires nothing more than your enhanced awareness of your inner healing force, the best part of you.

"Master, instruct me in the principles of the highest wisdom."

The teacher picked up his brush and painted one word: *"Attention."*

The student waited for more words to follow, but nothing came. "Is that all? Can you not tell me more?" he asked hastily.

The master again painted the same word twice: *"Attention. Attention."*

The student dismissed the advice as simple-minded and mundane and again requested more. The master responded, three times: *"Attention. Attention. Attention."*

Defensively the student asked, "What does that word *attention* mean anyway?" The sage answered gently, *"Attention means attention."*

Do not be misled by the outward simplicity of this prescription. Attention, the Zen master knows, is not easily cultivated and will elude even the most diligent student. When sleep does not come easily to me, my own efforts to focus on my personal bedtime story have been relentlessly interrupted by my worries and negative memories.

For example, once when reaching for sleep I began to recount my childhood story but immediately my narrative was interrupted by a painful memory. In a rash moment of five-year-old spite, I reached into my grandfather's jacket while his eyes were averted and took a handful of change to make my world more tolerable. It wasn't my grandfather's fault that I had to go to the dentist, and his money was only small compensation for the pain the dentist would inevitably inflict, but this seemed my only recourse to a morning of painful drilling and pulling.

Blast this memory! How will I ever get to sleep now? Before I left for the dentist each week, my grandfather would reach into that same jacket pocket filled with bills and coins to give me money for the dentist's bill. I easily blamed my pain on the man who paid the bill.

How will I ever get to sleep? Pay attention . . . pay attention . . . What a grueling morning. The anesthesia didn't work. The dentist seemed extra mean. The world of pain hovered over me like a dark cloud as

I stomped down the flights of stairs to the street and began my three-block walk back to our corner candy store.

Where is this memory coming from? Why now when I need to fall asleep? Pay attention . . . There was a silver lining, or so it seemed. The change from grandfather's pocket jingling in my own. I changed directions, headed toward the five-and-ten-cent store and dashed in when I was sure no one was looking. I headed straight to the lunch counter to commit a major act of heresy. I ordered a ham sandwich and Pepsi®, a luxury I not only could not afford but that broke the Kosher dietary laws I had been raised to believe were sacred. Yet secretly I had dreamed of a bite of the forbidden sandwich! With the ham and mustard I swallowed all of the warnings of what sin such an act would be!

I had completely forgotten this for almost half a century. Why is this memory revealing itself to me now when I really need to get some sleep? I wolfed the sandwich down in seconds, torn between not wanting to be caught and wanting to savor every forbidden bite. I downed my Pepsi® and for a brief moment forgot the pain of the dentist's drill. I felt vindicated as I made my way home with what would be my secret, forever.

Pay attention . . . I love myself . . . I did it . . . I went through it . . . but I love myself regardless . . . My moment of vindication was brief. Tragedy was waiting for me as soon as I walked in the door to my home. My grandfather was accusing my mother of stealing the missing change from his pocket. They were yelling. My mother denied it. My face must have told the entire story, because my grandfather turned to me the moment I walked in the door. Grandfather shook his finger at me, and as he yelled at me the veins in his hairless head bulged. Mother defended my five-year-old honor with such power and outrage that for the next three years I lived in the tiny apartment with two of the people I loved most in the world never speaking another word to each other. I suffered in fearful silence that the truth would be revealed. The silence in the house was so heavy. Soon I developed one inner ear infection after another, and if any words were to pass between my grandfather and my mother I would not have heard them because my hearing became so poor.

What a revelation! . . . Now it seemed clear as day to me why I had such a phobia of dentists, why for nearly forty years I would have rather suffered a toothache than visit a dentist. I knew the source of my ear infections and my mild hearing loss. I understood how my adult pain, no matter how much I sought to numb it, flared up into insomnia when I was under stress. I peered into a great cavern within my inner being, a deep crevice in my conscience. How would I ever fall asleep now?

I entreated myself to pay attention. I reminded myself over and over that no matter what I did, no matter what I went through, I certainly loved myself enough to let me get a good night's sleep. I sat upright in bed, reached for a pen and paper on my bedside, and wrote a note to myself: "My mother and grandfather have forgiven each other and they have long forgiven me. Now all that is left is for me to forgive myself." I woke, eight hours later, fully rested and at peace with myself. In the words of William Shakespeare: "He that sleeps feels not the toothache."

There is a Sufi aphorism that conveys the same feeling of contentment I experienced that morning: "When the heart weeps for what it has lost, the spirit laughs for what it has found."

Each person will experience different types and qualities of memories rushing to the forefront of their mind's stage. Some memories will be directly related to your personal story, and others will seemingly be quite scattered and unrelated. Jan was forty-five years of age and was suffering with insomnia for weeks before she came to see me. It was in the context of her case that I first shaped the Insomnia Wellness Rx presented to you now. Jan greeted the first night of her treatment with mixed relief and anxiety. She was a magnificently creative person and was looking forward to crafting her personal bedtime story.

When I arrived at my office the next morning at 8 A.M. there was already an answer on the phone machine. I pressed playback and heard Jan's excited voice on the tape. "Dr. Taub, this is Jan. It's 6 A.M. and I just had to call and tell you that I can sleep!" I called Jan back right away, a bit concerned that she was awake so early. Jan answered and was quick to tell me that she fell asleep within a half hour of crawling into bed at 9:30 P.M. She then described her personal bedtime story, which was based upon a memory of walking in the park with her mother when she was a little girl and her mother's laughter when they followed behind a parade of waddling ducks.

I asked Jan if she had any difficulty following her narrative. Indeed, at the beginning of her story, Jan's mind was interrupted by what seemed like an entirely unrelated grief-stricken memory. When her father died of cancer three years ago she wasn't with him to offer comfort or to say goodbye. She never stopped feeling guilty over this. As those pangs of guilt seemed on the verge of crawling into bed with her, she remembered her personal code of honor: "I will love myself no matter what I have done and no matter what I have been through." Jan consciously held on to this thought in her mind and was determined to do so until the feelings of guilt subsided. Before she could finish her bedtime story, the part where she and her mother hold the soft baby ducks in their hands, Jan was sound asleep.

Do not give up hope of sleep if your own personal bedtime story is interrupted by sorrowful or painful emotions and memories. Nights are not inhabited by dreams alone but also by strange thoughts that stir our souls and invite us to learn from them. Let the time before you fall asleep be an opportunity for distilling those harmful feelings and beliefs, the ones that are likely to contribute to illnesses and disease. Be merciful to yourself and let your personal bedtime story remind you of this mercy. In this way you can transform the painful quality of those emotions by wrapping them in the warm blanket of forgiveness and love. In *The Merchant of Venice*, a play about avarice, greed, and forgiveness, William Shakespeare described the nature and effect of mercy:

> *The quality of mercy is not strained,*
> *It droppeth as the gentle rain from heaven*
> *Upon the place beneath: it is twice blessed*
> *It blesseth him that gives and him that takes.*

Give mercy to yourself and you will be twice blessed—blessed first with a good night's sleep and blessed second with the forgiveness of painful memories. Every night when you go to sleep, consciously put your worries and painful memories to rest—forever. When your body, mind, and soul are at peace with your entire self, no disease, not even insomnia, can disrupt you. The Insomnia Wellness Rx will help you bring balance to your body, calmness to your mind, and peace to your soul. What more could you hope for from a good night's rest?

> *Hush! my dear, lie still and slumber,*
> *Holy angels guard thy bed!*
> *Heavenly blessing without number*
> *Gently falling on thy head.*
> —*Isaac Watts*, Divine Songs

WELLNESS RX FOR INSOMNIA

Make these promises in addition to the promises of the basic Wellness Rx summarized on page 108. For a lifetime of good night's sleep, follow these guidelines for one week and as necessary thereafter. Sign your name below.

1. *I promise to create a sleepy environment.*

2. *I promise to follow the therapeutic sleep routine.*

3. *I promise to put my worries to rest.*

4. *I promise to avoid uppers and downers.*

5. *I promise to eliminate unnecessary prescription drugs with my doctor's assistance.*

6. *I promise to tell myself a personal bedtime story.*

7. *I promise to establish a personal code of honor of honoring myself.*

8. *I promise to embrace the quality of mercy.*

_____

(your signature and today's date)

14

QUITTING SMOKING

It is not because things are difficult that we do not dare; it is because we do not dare that they are difficult.

—*Seneca*

Congratulations on choosing to save your life. By quitting smoking, you will allow the remarkable power of the Healing Force to reverse the entire damage to your body caused by smoking, as long as cancer or emphysema has not developed.

The Stop Smoking Wellness Rx integrates biomedical, psychological, and spiritual components to help you extinguish this addiction forever. The biomedical components will make your physical addiction to nicotine *easy* to conquer. All traces of nicotine will be eliminated from your system in less than seven days! In just one year, your risk of heart attack will decrease by 50 percent, and in time every other risk associated with smoking will be erased from your body.

The Stop Smoking Wellness Rx recognizes that there is much more to smoking than the physical addiction, and therefore any effort to quit forever cannot be restricted to the physical aspects of the addiction. The psychological and spiritual components of the Rx effectively neutralize the mental anguish associated with quitting as you learn the secret known to millions of ex-smokers: *once you make up your mind to quit, it is easy.*

Like many Americans, I have heard the Surgeon General's warnings about smoking, I have listened to the statistics on smoking-related illnesses, and I know that smoking is the single largest cause of death in this country—more than AIDS, automobile accidents, firearms, and alcohol, *combined.*

One would hope that these facts alone would encourage people to quit smoking. But clearly that has not generally been the case. Today, approximately sixty million adults in America smoke and more than three thousand children and teenagers start smoking *each day.* It is not clear whether these numbers are increasing or decreasing.

163

SAVE OUR CHILDREN

Although I have long encouraged my patients who smoke to quit, I only recently became impassioned about smoking cessation. Why? Because of all the new facts about the effects of secondhand smoke on children. As a pediatrician, and as a parent, I cannot ignore the fact that children living in households where parents smoke have 600 percent more respiratory and ear infections. It is reported that secondhand smoking triggers approximately 30,000 new cases of asthma and bronchitis in previously unaffected children and up to one million asthma attacks in children every year. Additionally, children who grow up in environments with cigarette smoke have growth problems, behavioral disorders, and tend to grow up to inherit their parents' addiction.

According to the Environmental Protection Agency, "passive smoking" contributes to up to 300,000 respiratory infections in infants alone each year, resulting in up to 15,000 hospitalizations annually. Individuals of all ages who are exposed to secondhand smoke are at least 30 percent more likely to develop cancer. Exposure to secondhand smoke is the third leading cause of death in the United States. Nationally, almost 150,000 women die each year of lung cancer caused by cigarettes. In my own practice, the mothers who smoked were twice as likely to develop lung cancer as their husbands who smoked. Trained and committed to protecting and fostering the good health of children, how could I ignore these findings?

I decided to conduct a demonstration project called "Save Our Children" in my small, community-based practice in Mount Carmel, California, where at least 80 percent of the sick children coming to see me smelled like stale smoke when I examined them. A recent local survey had indicated that over 50 percent of the schoolchildren in the community lived in homes where parents smoked.

Seventy parents made written promises to follow the Stop Smoking Wellness Rx described in this chapter for the sake of their children. Lederle Laboratories provided PROSTEP™ Nicotine Patches and technical assistance. When we first embarked on our project, I had no idea how much work it would demand of me. During prolonged and individual consultations, I heard each parent promise to quit smoking, a promise they made first to their children and then to God in whatever way their particular religious tradition inspired. Day and night, seven days a week, I educated, pleaded, counseled, coaxed, cajoled, and praised seventy nicotine-addicted parents who desperately wanted to free themselves, and their children, from the harmful effects of smoking. As an ex-smoker of fifteen years myself, I felt their cravings and experienced their triumphs. I exercised with them, ate with them, taught them yoga, and meditated and prayed with them.

What I learned from these dedicated parents is that smoking is much more than just a habit. Smoking is an overwhelmingly powerful addiction and a soul sickness. This addiction to nicotine, I learned, does much more than just destroy the body. It enslaves the mind and suppresses the soul. I discovered that nicotine addicts will do or say or promise *anything* to themselves, to their loved ones, and even to God if it gives them an excuse to *continue* smoking—often while pretending to quit. As I began to despair that the chains of nicotine addiction were unbreakable, I discovered part of the secret that I want to share with you: once you make up your mind to quit, nicotine addiction is one of the *easiest* addictions to overcome. Why? Because basically it is an addiction that is all in the mind. The physical withdrawal symptoms from nicotine addiction are actually very mild, tolerable, and short-lived. *It's the mental anguish that hurts the most.*

An astounding 95.6 percent of my patients quit smoking by the end of the six-week treatment program. You can quit too with the shorter and much simpler Stop Smoking Wellness Rx that I present in this chapter. This prescription is a reflection of my many years of professional experience with smoking patients as well as the massive clinical research performed at the nation's leading medical centers. The underlying principle of this treatment for smoking addiction is that the addiction itself is a symptom of a soul sickness. Any therapy that seeks permanent recovery from the addiction must address the mental, emotional, behavioral, and spiritual levels of the smoker. This treatment program is successful because it provides tools for healing addiction at every one of these levels.

JOIN THE 3500 AMERICANS WHO STOP SMOKING EACH DAY

If you want to join the thousands of people who quit smoking each day, you must first understand the true scope of the power that nicotine holds over you. Nicotine actually makes you believe that you cannot quit smoking even if you want to. When you become aware of this fact and literally see that this belief is all in your mind, you have already begun to break the chains of your addiction. The second fact to know is this: *quitting smoking is easy.* Once you get beyond the physical discomfort, which usually lasts less than a week even if you smoke one or two packs a day, the remaining obstacles are all in your mind. How much physical discomfort will you experience? You may experience some irritability, some nervousness, some sleeplessness, some dryness of the mouth, some forgetfulness, and certainly some cravings for cigarettes. The nicotine itself is out of your system in just three or four days after the last cigarette. The physical discomfort that you might experience is about at the misery level of a cold and a lot less than the flu.

How do I know that quitting is actually easy? I know it from thousands of patients who have told me so. "It was no problem once I made up my mind." If you ask an ex-smoker how he or she quit, the answer is virtually always the same: *once they made up their mind to quit, it was easy.* When I finally made up my mind to quit after smoking for twenty-five years, *it was easy.* My brother is also a physician, and he stopped smoking after twenty years. But it took two episodes of collapsed lungs and subsequent surgical procedures for him to make the commitment to quit. My brother actually smoked while recovering from surgery. He thought that he could just sneak a few puffs. Can you imagine how horrified the nurse was when she discovered smoke in the gallon jugs filled with water to which his chest tubes were connected? My brother now admits that once he made up his mind to stop, *it was easy.*

My stepfather tended bar and smoked for sixty years. He stopped immediately one day when at the age of seventy-eight he experienced an episode of slurred speech indicative of an impending stroke. Eight years later, he is perfectly healthy, claiming that once he made up his mind, *quitting was easy.* This a relief to our entire family, because statistics show that smokers have a 250 percent increase in stroke rates.

There is more to the secret of nicotine addiction. Statistics show that 90 percent of smokers want to quit but don't think they can. Remember that the nicotine has the power to make you believe that. But where else does this belief come from? In part it comes from the tobacco industry, which has helped cultivate the myth that once you start, the pleasure you get is so wonderful that quitting is just not worthwhile. It is obvious to see how this myth drives their company profits. They need to get you to buy only one pack and then you are hooked for life. What a deceitful and deathly advertising campaign. And the tobacco companies will stop short of nothing to get their messages out there. Marlboro recently foiled network television's restrictions against cigarette advertisements by erecting an enormous billboard just beyond the gate of a national ballpark, always in view of the cameras looking out over the field from home plate.

Light Up Your Energy, Not a Cigarette!

What the tobacco industry overlooks and would like to cover up is the fact that even the most heavily addicted smoker has a natural instinct for self-preservation, an instinct that is more powerful than anything the tobacco companies can devise. This instinct is the calling of your inner Healing Force. In fact, the Healing Force, or what science calls homeostasis, is the key to quitting smoking. And it is a force far too sophisticated and powerful for the smoking industry to comprehend. Homeostasis is dedicated to keeping your energy in balance and recognizes the harm done to this balance by cigarettes. This Stop Smoking Wellness Rx will help you ignite your Healing Force to overcome your addiction to smoking. The process of recharging your homeostasis to triumph over cigarettes is called the *De-addiction Process.*

   Your instinct for self-preservation has been suppressed not only by the smoke you inhale and the nicotine absorbed into your blood but also by the universal smoker's belief that "it's just too tough to quit." Where does this belief come from? It is a dangerous joke played on you by the tobacco industry. I call it a joke because of the smiles on the faces of the tobacco company executives whose profits skyrocket as your health plummets. Half a million American smokers die each year while tobacco company executives get wealthier and wealthier. Tobacco industry lawyers and representatives speak of "smokers' rights." Who's right are they really talking about? The right to go out and buy a pack of cigarettes? What none of these lawyers want to talk about is the implicit right being defended here to slowly kill themselves and make their children sick. What they are really defending is their right to make a profit off of your self-destruction. Why do tobacco companies employ so many lawyers? Perhaps because they are lying when they claim that smoking does not cause lung cancer. How can the tobacco companies not feel responsibility for the fact that 17 percent of third- to sixth-grade children are smokers?

Murderous Myths

Tobacco companies spend 6.5 million dollars each and every day to gain new nicotine addicts *and* to keep reminding you and other nicotine addicts how enjoyable it is to smoke. As a nicotine addict, you have been convinced that smoking gives you pleasure. You have suppressed the fact that you are really just *dependent* on the chemical called nicotine so as not to feel badly *without* it. That is entirely different from the chemical giving you pleasure. The actual pleasure you may have received from smoking came a long time ago, at the very beginning of your addiction. Now you have to smoke to just not feel bad, and that's a big difference from the enjoyment myth the tobacco companies promote. Unfortunately, the myth has an inescapable conclusion for you: "If my cigarettes are so enjoyable, why should I stop and make myself feel so bad?" The success of the enjoyment myth is measured by the half-million Americans who lose their lives to it each year. More American lives are lost to this myth in just twelve months than were lost during all of the years of the Vietnam War.

The myth of enjoyment is bolstered by the myth of how physically difficult it is to quit smoking. The actual physical discomfort of nicotine withdrawal is minimal and short-lived. It nevertheless receives the majority of attention from consumers, doctors, drug companies, and other commercial interests.

I recently did some work with prison inmates who had their smoking privileges taken away. Many unexpected outcomes emerged. I prescribed nicotine patches for the inmates to gradually eliminate their addiction to nicotine. The patches are generally recommended at full strength for a month and half strength for another month. I was totally surprised, however, that once the inmates knew they had no choice but to quit they hardly noticed any physical discomfort. In three or four days most requested a reduction in the patches to just half strength, and a few days later they were no longer interested in the patches at all.

Cigarettes Are Not for the Soul

If you are addicted to nicotine, your body is at *dis-ease*. In this case, ILL is clearly equivalent to I Lack Love. Science without soul has provided very little practical assistance for smokers, or for that matter, addicts of any substance, because it fails to see addiction in these crucial terms. One of the major reasons for the success of Alcoholics Anonymous is the organization's openness to matters of the soul and its commitment to addressing the mental, emotional, physical, and spiritual aspects of addiction.

Addressing the addiction to smoking at the level of the soul means opening up the soul to a healing intervention. The most successful strategy for healing nicotine addiction is to actually de-medicalize the treatment plan. The Stop Smoking Wellness Rx does this by adopting the Serenity Prayer as part of a spiritual component to treatment that is just as important, indeed more important, than any traditional biological or medical components. The Serenity Prayer is powerful because it recognizes a Higher Power or God that constantly offers healing and grace to those who turn toward that Power. Part of overcoming an addiction to smoking entails turning toward, rather than away from, a Higher Power.

The power of nicotine to keep you from accepting that Higher Power of healing is fierce. Nicotine convinces your brain that it can counteract unhappiness, depression, angst, existential suffering, and even loss of faith. Your inner works have been broken by the force of nicotine, and certainly no cigarette is going to heal them. We all carry our scars with us, but unlike most scars, the scar of smoking won't fade with time unless you actively determine to overcome nicotine's power by igniting the Healing Force within you. That is the only force capable of surpassing and containing the power of nicotine over your mind.

Joe Camel Isn't Cool, He's a Killer

People who began smoking thirty years ago started for different reasons than baby boomers smoking today. They were drawn in by the new magic of television and its images of the good life. Cigarettes were recommended by doctors who actually recommended certain brands for different ailments. People then watched Humphrey Bogart and Lauren Bacall fill the giant silver screens of their childhood, with cigarettes dangling between their movie-star lips. And who could forget the Marlboro mechanic who looked up from the car engine he was repairing just long enough to tell you: "It's good for you to smoke while you are working."

Individuals today start smoking because their parents did and because of stress, insecurity, depression, anxiety, hopelessness, violence, and relentless peer group pressure. Women are told that they've come a long way and if they smoke they will go even farther. Kids think that Joe Camel is cool. Researchers suggest that the popularity of the Joe Camel image is a major influence on the massive numbers of children who start smoking every day. The company that produces Camels refuses to see the tragedy in this and claims that Joe Camel is merely designed to attract smokers away from competing brands. Once again our favorite television shows are linking cigarettes to wealth, success, and glamour. In a recent survey, one-quarter of over a hundred popular shows portrayed high-profile, successful, role-model type actors and actresses engaged in smoking.

You have been led to believe that you need tremendous willpower to quit smoking. This belief is entirely backward. Quitting smoking doesn't require willpower. Quite the opposite, to stop smoking requires that you stop *using* your willpower to smoke. As a smoker, you *use* your willpower to go to the store, then to buy your cigarettes, then to take them out of the pack, then to light them, then to inhale. You must stop using your willpower to smoke. The only force greater than your will to smoke is your Healing Force, if only you can ignite it. This Stop Smoking Wellness Rx will show you how to do just that.

People who continue to smoke while realizing that they are destroying their health and potentially the health of those around them usually explain their behavior in one or all of these ways:

- I smoke for pleasure.
- I don't think I can stop.
- I don't want to gain weight.

It is actually the nicotine addiction itself that is talking! The nicotine addiction is so powerful that it literally has a life and a will of its own and will promote thoughts and beliefs, no matter how false, just to avoid being extinguished. Even though it has been fifteen years since I last smoked a cigarette, I still vividly recall the pleasure smoking seemed to provide in my life. After I quit I used to wake up startled and in a sweat, three or four times a year, from a dream that I had broken down and smoked again. This dream recurred for ten years. Now, finally, I don't dream that dream at all. But for ten years the power of nicotine lingered in my sleepy mind.

Would I ever smoke again? Never! Would I smoke if I were in the middle of a war; if I were fleeing from a ravaged country; if I were experiencing the worst type of pain, suffering, or deprivation I could imagine? Never! My addiction is entirely healed.

Roots of Addiction

What does the infant do from the moment of birth? It sucks on thumbs, nipples, blanket corners, fists, toys, pacifiers, and just about anything that will fit inside a tiny mouth. The actual embryo even begins to thumbsuck at four months' gestation. At birth the infant frantically roots, screaming for oral contact. Not finding a nipple, the infant latches on to a thumb. You don't have to be a Freudian to recognize that the *overriding* characteristic of a human infant is the oral urge and the instinct and reflex to suck.

In the psychological and emotional life of an infant, pleasure comes to be viewed in terms of this instinctual desire to suck on something. Depending significantly on how the sucking urge has been fulfilled, infant and toddler development proceeds through an Oedipal stage, a homosexual phase, and usually to a heterosexual orientation. If the infant grows up in an environment surrounded by tobacco smells, it may associate those smells with pleasure forever. If the growing baby becomes emotionally stressed with feelings of neglect, abandonment, or fear, as babies often do in their new and uncertain world, the earlier oral phase of existence typically reemerges in a craving for oral pleasure that can lead to overeating and habits of a sucking nature. Smoking becomes a remembrance of things past elicited by warm feelings on the palate and sensations of fullness in the back of the throat.

Indeed, research indicates that what smokers seek to access through a good, long "hit" is not so much the feeling of fullness in the lungs or the increase in blood nicotine levels but rather the congested, scratchy, irritating *but warm feeling,* experienced on the palate and in back of the throat. Smokers continue to smoke for the feeling of security they experienced when sucking as a child. If the security basis of addiction is not dealt with, the potential for relapse will persist forever. Therefore, the Stop Smoking Wellness Rx has been developed to direct you to the ultimate source of your self-healing: your own inner Healing Force, homeostasis. The Rx helps you turn to the authentic source of security that lies within you rather than relying on the false promises of external pleasures.

BEGINNING THE END OF ADDICTION

Smokers become slaves to cigarettes because they yearn for pleasure and security. They puff away, trying to satisfy oral needs and regain warm and fuzzy feelings they experienced in childhood. They have been tricked into believing that smoking can provide that warmth and security. They have been addicted.

The beginning of the end of smoking starts when you recognize the worthlessness of these statements: "I don't think I'll ever smoke again." "I'll try to stop." "I'm pretty sure I can." The end of smoking occurs when you finally flick on the internal switch in your mind that declares: "I am no longer a smoker and I will never smoke again."

All statements beginning with *I'll try* need to be replaced with the declarative *I will.* How do you get from *I'll try* to *I will?* It is only possible to get from here to there through the following:

- Enhancing self-esteem
- Awakening personal power
- Recognizing and confronting fears
- Establishing personal responsibility, self-value, and reverence for life

More things are accomplished through personal power and prayer than this world currently imagines. This De-addiction Process allows you to gain the physical energy needed to overcome nicotine addiction, the mental ability to finally reject it, and the spiritual power to heal it forever.

The problem really isn't with stopping smoking. The real problem is discovering how not to start again. The only sure way of preventing relapse is *healing* the addiction. More than a decade of personal and clinical experience with patients has gone into developing this Rx for de-addiction. I started with myself fifteen years ago when I decided to quit a three-pack-a-day habit cultivated for twenty-five years. I was overweight, had tension headaches, and chronic bronchitis, and *craved* the feeling that nicotine seemed to provide. What made me so determined to quit?

I was standing over an autopsy table peering into the open chest cavity of a patient who had just died from lung cancer. He was a physician, a colleague, just fifty-three years of age with a wife, three children, and healthy parents. I grew lightheaded as I observed the sheer destruction of the entire inside of his body. It was possible to see the damage caused by the three packs of cigarettes he smoked daily for forty years. I thought of my own father, whom I had adored. Ever since the time I was just three or four years old, I remember him with a cigarette in his mouth, chain smoking and with yellowed and stained fingertips. He also died at fifty-three with heart and lung disease.

Standing there at the autopsy table, I looked down at my yellowed and stained fingers and realized that I was much more like my father than I had ever imagined. And then I pictured my own children, so beautiful and full of life. Did I want them to grow up to be just like me? I knew instantly that my smoking habit was over. I quit smoking ten days later, January 1, 1978.

But my own story is not the only triumph over smoking, and it is admittedly more dramatic and graphic than most people's experiences. Let me tell you about one of the heroes of Mount Carmel who quit smoking to save his life.

A SUCCESS STORY

My patient, Johnny Hoffman, grew up on a farm near Mount Carmel and worked as a coal miner. He appeared to me to be a heart attack just ready to happen or a lung just ready to collapse when I first saw him in my office. As if the mines did not put enough strain on his lungs, Johnny was a heavy smoker, a habit he shared with his wife. They both agreed to embark on the Stop Smoking Wellness Rx, which they completed with tremendous success. The following transcript is from a visit six months after Johnny quit smoking. His lungs sounded remarkably clear and the years of smoking left barely an audible mark.

"I forget. How old are you, Johnny?"

"I'll be fifty this fall, Doctor."

"When did you start to smoke?"

"When I was a freshman in junior college. I was about seventeen or eighteen and started to smoke religiously like the other guys to just look cool; you know how it is. I even met my future wife then, and she started smoking with me. I quit three or four times since, but each time I came back. I was over three packs a day when I came to you, Doctor. This forty-dollar-a-week habit was breaking me. I think the fact we were out on strike and I needed money, combined with how bad you told me my lungs sounded, was the straw that broke the camel's back."

"Did you do anything special when you quit before?"

"Nope. Except the one time I quit for seven months, which was the last time I quit, I was hypnotized. That worked for awhile I guess, and I didn't even have any withdrawal symptoms. But this Wellness Rx has really been a very successful deal. Margaret and I were just sitting around last night talking about how clean we smell and how great we feel. The kids don't cough, and their noses aren't snotty all the time any more.

"I don't know, though. I came to you originally because I wanted you to give me the nicotine patch, not all this 'wellness stuff.' But I know that I didn't really need the patch. I stopped it in less than a week anyway. I just needed the change in lifestyle to feel better. I get on my treadmill and walk at the rate of ten to twelve kilometers an hour too, which is clipping along pretty good. I don't even get tired. I also started parking in the far parking lot at work and walk a quarter of a mile to and from my car." Johnny lifted up his foot to show me the treads on a new pair of Rockport® walking shoes.

"You and Margaret are remarkable."

"I don't know what happened to me, but I sure am really feeling great."

"What medications were you on?"

"Tenormin and a diuretic called hydrochlorthiazide. But I haven't taken either medicine for the last two months now. What's my pressure?"

"115 over 75. It's like a teenager, Johnny."

"I feel like one. My kids say I act like one."

"How long had you been hypertensive?"

"Since I was thirty years old at least. When I came to see you last spring it was 150 over 98. You jumped on me pretty good for that."

"I remember."

"I threw away my cigarettes forever."

"Refresh my memory about your change in lifestyle, please."

"Well, my day used to be that I would wake up . . . but first of all I smoked all night long. At least every two hours I would wake up and I would smoke.

"Next I would stumble into the bathroom and smoke in there, just waiting to really wake up. Then during the drive to work between Allendale and Owensville I would probably smoke about ten cigarettes before I got to the cafe near the mine. Every morning I ate two eggs, sausage, and hashbrowns and three or four cups of coffee. I smoked about a half a pack with breakfast just shooting the breeze with everyone before the morning whistle blew.

"Then I smoked all the time at work, not actually in the mine itself, of course, but every free minute outside of the mine I lit up. At lunch I ate fast-food hamburgers with double cheese. At night Margaret usually made a good meat-and-potatoes-type meal. I smoked after dinner, I smoked watching television, and when I finally went to sleep, I smoked every two hours because I'd wake up."

"And now? How is your lifestyle different now?"

"I'm up early in the morning to exercise and meditate. Actually though, I have to tell you that the first week I wasn't supposed to smoke in the house, I cheated a little bit and smoke in the attached garage. Then the next week I sneaked just two puffs in my truck on the way to work. It all just came together for me the next week. For the both of us.

"I still go to the cafe for breakfast every morning during the week, but I have a bowl of hot oatmeal, two pieces of whole-wheat toast without butter, and decaffeinated coffee. On weekends, Margaret usually makes us fresh muffins or maybe buys some bagels. For lunch I have a big salad and some hearty whole-wheat bread. For dinner Margaret usually cooks something with rice or pasta. We both love Chinese food, and Margaret is using a wok a lot. We eat rice with chicken instead of pork or beef, but only once or twice a week. Margaret was the one who bought the treadmill. I use it every day. I feel great."

"How is your weight, Johnny?"

"I started the Wellness Rx at 225 pounds and my cholesterol was 280. You said that was pretty outrageous. I gotta tell you that didn't make me feel good. Well, I weighed myself just last week and now I'm at 198 pounds."

"Twenty-seven pounds in six months is pretty great."

"I just stuck to the high rungs on the food ladder and got at least twenty minutes of exercise every day, like you said. What is my cholesterol now?"

"It's down to 170, and your HDL and LDL are within normal limits. I'm really proud of you, Johnny."

"I'm proud of me too."

Just Make Up Your Mind

Tens of millions of ex-smokers understand that you can quit only when you have truly made up your mind to do so. That decision alone has taken some ex-smokers years to come to! But it is really not so difficult to make up your mind when you consider the facts and not just what the tobacco advertisements want you to believe. Remember that physical withdrawal symptoms stop in less than a week and any misery you experience after the first seven days is entirely in your mind. That's good news since you have already learned several tools for cultivating health-inspiring and energy-creating thoughts and beliefs to replace those that invite illness and defend harmful habits.

The De-addiction Process extinguishes your addiction by balancing your body, mind, and spirit through stimulating your own natural Healing Force. Thousands of laboratory experiments and controlled observations of human behavior demonstrate how we can use our thoughts, feelings, and attitudes to overcome addictions. I have described the power of your natural Healing Force as equivalent to the presence of God in each and every one of your trillions of cells. To unleash this Healing Force, you must first quiet your mind and let your thoughts become like a quiet ocean instead of a raging river. When your thoughts are rarely ever still, nicotine just stirs them up even more as the chemical unsettles and disrupts your mind and suffocates your spirit.

To understand your addiction, and in turn to understand how to disempower it, first recall that your body is energy. When your energy is balanced, you are generally well. The introduction of a foreign chemical like the nicotine molecule disrupts and short-circuits your energy system. The chemical structure of nicotine is so foreign to your own energy that it causes your system to become out of balance and ill. To accommodate that foreign energy, three things typically occur in your body:

1. *Dependence.* To counteract the imbalance and to overcome the disruption of natural energy, your body actually incorporates the foreign chemical energy of nicotine and then gradually grows to need the nicotine to just not feel bad. This is the first stage of addiction. The dependence factor causes your body to unnaturally rely on the drug to just not feel bad and programs your thoughts to demand the drug. You become hooked and then you smoke not to feel good but to just avoid feeling bad.

2. *Tolerance.* Slowly but surely your energy system begins to require more and more nicotine just to achieve the same feeling of "not feeling bad." The onset of this stage will vary according to your body size and other physiological factors. A half pack of cigarettes a day quickly escalates to one or two packs because your system needs more and more nicotine to just not feel bad. Increasing amounts of nicotine are required just to satisfy the dependence factor.

3. *Withdrawal.* The third and final stage of the addiction process is the development of the withdrawal factor. You experience distress, discomfort, and disease when you deprive your system of that foreign energy because your energy system has actually come to depend on nicotine just to not feel bad. You feel physically ill when the nicotine is not provided. You feel withdrawn. But the actual experience of withdrawal is not as physically tortuous as you have been led to believe. When you become addicted, your nicotine-drenched thoughts block your natural Healing Force that would otherwise attempt to break the addiction. Your thoughts tell you it is too enjoyable to give

up nicotine and that it would be too difficult and uncomfortable to stop even if you really wanted to. When you are addicted to nicotine, you become powerless to just casually *think* your way out of the addiction. You must therefore make up your mind to stop, set a quitting date, and then begin relying on a much more powerful force to get you through the De-addiction Process—the Healing Force. Because your smoke-stained thoughts have actually been programmed to support, maintain, justify, rationalize, and defend your addiction *at all costs,* you cannot expect these same thoughts to help you to decide to quit.

The Stop Smoking Wellness Rx is based upon three principles:

- You can't fight an addiction to nicotine with nicotine-drenched thoughts.
- You must surrender to a Higher Power, God, to ignite the natural Healing Force capable of breaking the powerful chains of nicotine addiction.
- You must have faith and demonstrate love.

Your Physician's Role

The Stop Smoking Wellness Rx is a complement to the powerful help that your physician can provide while you quit smoking. Statistics indicate very clearly that there is no more powerful incentive to convince smokers to quit than a physician's encouragement and warning. In almost all instances, physicians will refer their motivated patients to local programs for help, and if requested they will offer their patients a form of nicotine replacement therapy with nicotine skin patches or nicotine gum.

Forms of nicotine replacement therapy that are presently available can be quite effective for about 10 percent of smokers, but only when combined with a comprehensive behavior modification strategy. Such therapy is essentially worthless without guidelines for changing personal behavior. A nicotine patch or gum does not make the smoker want to quit; the patches and gum simply provide a crutch to help allay some physical withdrawal symptoms and mental cravings. However, the smoker's nicotine-drenched thoughts talk him or her into expecting that the patches or gum will make up their minds for them, and they usually abandon their behavior modification program.

The major problem with nicotine replacement therapy is that the patient spends so much time and energy on what the patch or gum is doing physically that he or she may play down or ignore the mental and spiritual aspects of the addiction. Nicotine patch wearers or nicotine gum chewers tend to enter an almost compulsive mental framework and dwell on:

- how the new nicotine drug makes them feel
- the rashes, nervousness, headaches, and nightmares they may experience
- whether their dose is too much, too little, or just right
- when the therapy should stop
- what will happen when the therapy is stopped

Used in conjunction with a program for changing personal lifestyle, nicotine replacement therapy can provide a temporary crutch to a significant percentage of patients who want to quit. Some of the new developments on the horizon, particularly a nicotine spray or inhaler, may add an additional level of therapeutic effectiveness. The irritation these substances cause to the actual tissues of the palate and throat may be more likely to satisfy the sucking reflex and instinct and the smoker's attempt to satisfy that need.

The larger issue with replacement therapy is the fact that it concentrates almost entirely on lessening the physical withdrawal symptoms to decrease the mental cravings of the smoker. This is a circuitous pathway, which is not necessarily a bad thing for some smokers who might benefit if they stay with a behavior modification strategy, and if they can afford the expense. The real problem with replacement therapy, however, is that the mental cravings of the smoker are not just a function of physical withdrawal symptoms. The cravings are much more a reflection of the misery that the media and tobacco industry have programmed the consumer's mind to expect and they also reflect a lack of self-esteem.

Nicotine addiction is an illness, and although nicotine replacement therapy "medicalizes" the cure, patients tend to invest it with unreasonable expectations. Patches or nicotine gum may diminish the sense of personal responsibility, enabling (and enobling!) the addict to shield him- or herself from the effects of loneliness, frustration, and worry that cigarettes are being used to mask in the first place.

The addictive personality generally begins in very early childhood, when the developing ego becomes disturbed and disrupted. The addictive person often grows up with very high expectations and without the ability to realize those expectations. Addictiveness in adult life tends to be a mental defense against a deep-seated lack of self-esteem. By all means, speak with your physician about quitting smoking and discuss the potential benefits of nicotine replacement therapy. Just remember that you don't absolutely *need* it and that once you make up your mind, *quitting smoking is easy.*

The vast majority of smokers find that their efforts are significantly enhanced by the help and presence of a physician who is willing to support their endeavor. It is important for physicians to be aware that smoking is not purely or even largely a physical addiction. Smoking is mostly a reflection of an uneasy soul, a soul sickness. Any therapy that seeks to effect lasting recovery from the addiction must address the emotional, behavioral, and spiritual levels of an individual's addiction.

Come now. Balance your energy to unleash your natural Healing Force. Your permanent de-addiction from smoking can begin only when:

- You make a meaningful declaration to quit.
- You choose a specific quit date.
- You make a vow to quit forever.
- You promise to take personal responsibility to keep your vow.

The De-addiction Process itself has built-in motivational factors that will encourage, support, and empower you to quit smoking. The process itself stimulates hope, and where there is personal hope, there is personal power to create long-term healing and change. You should not be at all discouraged if you have tried to stop smoking and failed. Even if they did not promote lasting change, your prior efforts have set you on the path to de-addiction. You now have a head start. It has been statistically proven that each time you attempt to stop smoking you get that much closer to success. It has been said, after all, that saints are sinners who never gave up. Many ex-smokers are smokers who *gave up.*

Keep in mind that becoming addicted to nicotine in the first place took you years and years—the roots of smoking addiction began to grow deep in your mind and body even before you actually started to smoke. They began to take hold in your mind when as an infant you were surrounded by smoke, you observed your parents smoke, or you saw attractive, wealthy people on television smoking. There has never been a more important time for you to stop smoking than now, because the latest news suggests that each cigarette brings you at least seven minutes closer to your death. One in every five deaths in this country is directly caused by cigarettes.

Your nicotine-addicted mind may be telling you that you just *can't* free yourself from this habit. That is understandable. It is understandable because the smoking addiction *itself* is causing your mind's repetition of those thoughts. You *think* they are your thoughts, but they are the nicotine-drenched thoughts of your addiction trying to keep itself alive. You have the capacity to change your thoughts once you are aware that it is the nicotine itself that is actually making your mind produce the thought that you *need* to keep smoking. You have the power to uproot those thoughts and weed out the harmful addiction. The discomfort of quitting is so much less than your nicotine-addicted mind can imagine.

"As you think, so you are." It is important for you to begin to think like a nonsmoker. Any hesitations you feel, any fears you experience, any ambivalence about quitting comes from the mind of a smoker. If you think like a smoker, you will continue to be a smoker. The De-addiction Process begins to neutralize your harmful smoker's thoughts. Meditation will further this process, as will your good behavior, because these activities cultivate new and healthful thought patterns. One of the most effective ways to heal a harmful habit is by replacing it with a health-promoting habit. It took you a long time to learn to smoke (no one gets the inhale right the first time), so don't expect to learn how not to smoke overnight. Have patience.

Like an overgrown garden, the process of uprooting weedlike thoughts and belief patterns cannot be completed in a day. Positive, "health-full" habits will take time to cultivate. That is why this program lasts for three weeks. But the results will last a lifetime.

Take pride in your decision to light up your life instead of a cigarette. Honor yourself and your soul for being courageous enough to begin the process of de-addiction. Self-pride and honor are potent healers. As you begin this process, remember:

- keep a distance from smokers or smoky places
- to watch your thoughts
- that smoking does not make you a lesser person
- that smoking will never satisfy your longings

Become Fearless

The vast majority of smokers want to stop, but two basic fears prevent them from doing so:

- the fear of failure
- the fear of gaining weight

If you are gripped by the fear of failure, remember that the fear of failure itself can lead to failure more quickly than can real efforts. To detach yourself from this fear so that it cannot sabotage your efforts to stop smoking, you will be reciting the Serenity Prayer that has been a part of Alcoholics Anonymous for decades. This simple nondenominational prayer has been a powerful source of strength and healing for millions of addicted people. The prayer has a spiritual magic about it that is quite beyond description but has to do with surrendering to a Higher Power. There will simply be no reason for failure or fearing failure with this newly kindled faith regardless of how you personally define or envision that Higher Power.

> *God grant me the serenity to accept the things I cannot change,*
> *the courage to change the things that I can,*
> *and the wisdom to know the difference.*
>
> *—Reinhold Niebuhr*

Recite this lovely prayer standing or sitting in front of a mirror and look into your own eyes. You may wish to add a prayer that has particular meaning to you.

I understand the fear of failure. I experienced it myself when I quit smoking. I was quitting for my children's sake. I was terrified by the thought that if I failed to quit, I failed them. The Stop Smoking Wellness Rx extinguishes that fear by replacing it with faith in yourself as well as faith in a Higher Power. It is crucial that you follow the Rx exactly as written for the necessary energy to break the chains of your addiction. Follow every single one of the Rx's components. Your nicotine addiction will do anything possible to defend itself, particularly when confronted with its imminent demise. The first thing the addiction will do is try to convince you to break one of the seven simple promises of the Rx—usually the exercise portion. When you recognize the addiction for what is, when you declare your power over it, nothing will stand in the way of your healing process.

You Don't Have to Gain Weight to Be Smoke-free

Most smokers say that they fear weight gain so much that it is just not worth quitting. This is the nicotine addiction talking again. There is a tendency to gain weight, but the average person only gains four pounds. When you consider the fact that each cigarette propels you seven minutes closer to death, four pounds is pretty inconsequential. However, even this minimal weight gain can be avoided by following the Wellness Rx nutrition guidelines. Especially if you stay on the upper rungs of the ladder, among the fruits, vegetables, and complex carbohydrates, your body will continue to burn excess fat, and even giving up your cigarettes will not cause you to gain weight.

THE CRAVING IS GONE IN TWENTY SECONDS

Keep in mind always that any discomfort you feel after five or six days will be purely mental, not physical—just a fleeting thought, an old desire, a passing craving, the last gasps of a dying habit. The De-addiction Process gives you the tools for disempowering these mental cravings by providing large doses of what the soul craves: love, forgiveness, faith, honor, esteem. Overcome the addiction's craving by practicing deep breathing, say the Serenity Prayer to yourself, or just remind yourself until the craving passes that it is all in your mind. If you do these things you will not break down and smoke. Your mental cravings and impulses won't last more than twenty seconds or so. Not much time to give up in exchange for a lifetime of renewed health, vitality, and energy.

Now, if you are ready to be free of your addiction to nicotine and cigarettes, begin the following week-by-week, step-by-step program for de-addiction. The guidelines listed contain the components of the Wellness Rx described in Chapter Eleven but in addition include smoking-specific strategies for stomping out your addiction to cigarettes and for lighting up your natural Healing Force.

THE STOP SMOKING WELLNESS RX: THE DECLARATION WEEK

The first stage of permanent smoking cessation involves a personal, sincere, and heartfelt declaration to quit. The specific requirements of this week are not difficult to fulfill. In fact, you are not even required to quit smoking *this* week. Right now, the most important thing you must do is declare to quit *one week* from today.

This week lays the groundwork for quitting smoking once and for all, so follow these guidelines carefully and completely so that you will have a solid foundation for quitting. Before beginning, you must be sure that you have first signed the Wellness Rx on page 108.

The Stop Smoking Wellness Rx rests upon the seven promises of the general Wellness Rx that you signed on page 108. In addition to those seven promises, the Stop Smoking Wellness Rx requires your promise to do the following:

- Recite the Serenity Prayer out loud and in front of a mirror each morning for the next seven days. Do this before you have breakfast or your first cup of coffee.

  God grant me the serenity to accept the things I cannot change, the courage to change the things I can, and the wisdom to know the difference.

  You may also wish to recite a prayer that is especially meaningful to you in the context of your own religious or spiritual beliefs. After reciting the prayer, take a moment or two to record a personal note or feeling in a journal, diary, or the blank page at the end of this chapter.

- It is not absolutely necessary, but *try* to cut in half the number of cigarettes you normally smoke. Also, *try* to delay your first morning cigarette until after you shower, shave or put on your makeup, and finish your breakfast. *This is the only optional promise on this list.*

- Smoke *only* outdoors this week. Do not smoke in your house, not even in the garage. If it is cold, then just dress warmly. Throw away every ashtray in the house immediately.

- Save all of your cigarette butts in a jar with some water at the bottom. A baby food jar is the perfect size to carry with you to work. This will be a constant reminder of what used to go into your lungs.

- Agree to have your last cigarette forever, by midnight, seven days from the moment you flush away your regular cigarettes. Throw away your lighters, no matter how expensive. Don't harm someone else by supporting their smoking addiction.

  I hereby vow on my honor and integrity that I will quit smoking exactly seven days from today.

  _____

  (your signature and today's date)

THE WITHDRAWAL WEEK

The first day of this week is your first nonsmoking day. Congratulations! Keep your butt jar handy to gaze at or for a sniff whenever you feel a strong craving for a cigarette. Keep following the promises you made last week. If you slip up on a promise, forgive yourself and just keep going on with a renewed commitment and responsibility.

Continue to keep the seven basic promises of the Wellness Rx. Additionally, promise to add these next five components to your Rx:

- Recite the Serenity Prayer every day
- Practice random acts of kindness every day
- Practice breathing techniques and simple yoga every day
- Make environmental changes
- Make behavior changes

Let's look at these new promises closely. They are so simple but must not be overlooked.

Random Acts of Kindness

Promise to commit one random act of kindness each and every day this week. A college professor in California gave his students this same assignment to compensate for all the random acts of violence that they were studying about. The students were encouraged to be as imaginative, spontaneous, and senseless as possible in their acts of caring and charity. One young man bought blankets from the Salvation Army and gave them to a group of homeless people gathered under a bridge. That didn't take a lot of time or a lot of money, but just imagine how much nicer the world could be if everyone did something like that. Now, imagine how much nicer you would feel about *yourself* if you did something like that every day.

One student pulled out of a parking space that she had just occupied and allowed a frantic student who was clearly late for class to park there instead. Another student encountered a homeless father and son at a convenience store and bought them several items of food. Don't even bother to contemplate your own acts of kindness, charity, and caring this week. The more spontaneous, the better.

I asked the editor of the Mount Carmel newspaper to fax me the Associated Press article about these college students, and he wrote across the top of the fax: "Dear Doctor. Here's the article. If there is ever anything else that I can do to help your research, please let me know." That was a random act of kindness. Opportunities for kindness exist wherever you are and whatever you do, especially with the elderly or ill. On the phone, on the bus, at work, in school, at church, while shopping, at home, through the mail. The potential for kindness in any of these places is unlimited.

Your random acts of kindness will reveal wonders and surprises for you as they open the doors for you to view yourself with more esteem and worth. You will grow with each experience. Whatever lies behind you or ahead of you is a tiny matter compared with what lies within you. Mother Teresa once commented that so many people are suffering from the lack of just some ordinary bread and ordinary love and kindness. Especially the very elderly could use some of your compassion today. As an ex-smoker now, you can do so much for others and yourself.

> *A man can only do what he can do.*
> *But if he does that each day*
> *he can sleep at night*
> *and do it again the next day.*
>
> *—Albert Schweitzer*

Proper Breathing and Simple Yoga

Promise to do the very simple yoga postures and breathing exercises described fully in Chapter Seven every single day this week. Do this in addition to, *not instead of,* the aerobic exercise you choose to do this week. The yoga and breathing take about fifteen or twenty minutes a day. Yoga, breathing, exercise, and meditation require *altogether* about sixty minutes of your time each day. Not bad when you consider that just nine cigarettes bring you more than sixty minutes closer to the end of your life.

Change Your Environment

Don't invite smokers to your house unless they agree not to smoke. This *includes* your parents, your children, your best friends. Decline any invitations to smokers' houses. Change your car pool if someone is smoking, or if necessary just plead with or bribe the person not to smoke. Avoid smoky places like bars and certain restaurants. At this stage of quitting smoking, it is crucial for you to keep in mind that your environment can be stronger than your will because of the power of nicotine. If smoking is allowed in your workplace, please photocopy this note and give it to your employer:

To the Employer of This Patient:

I am the physician helping the bearer of this letter in a very serious Stop Smoking effort. I respectfully request that you make a humane as well as sensible decision to ban smoking in this person's workplace. The decision is clearly humane because agencies of the United States government have declared that secondhand smoke causes sinusitis, respiratory infections, emphysema, and lung cancer. The decision is eminently sensible too because it is only a matter of time until employers become legally and financially responsible for the illnesses occurring in employees as a result of smoking being allowed in the workplace.

Thank you very much for your consideration in this urgent matter.

Sincerely,
Edward A. Taub, M.D.

Change Your Behavior

- Drink at least six glasses of water daily.
- Whenever you speak on the phone, transfer the phone to your other ear instead of the one you usually choose. Smokers miss smoking when on the phone, and this move confuses the addiction and lessens the craving.
- After you have seated yourself comfortably in your car, move at least eight inches to the left. Smokers have a very clear ritual for entering their car and placing themselves at a perfect distance from the ashtray. This move confuses the addiction and lessens the craving.
- Suck on a stick of black licorice or a cinnamon stick, or chew some gum right after you finish eating if you experience any cravings. Smokers associate finishing a meal with smoking a cigarette, and this will help dissolve the strong connection.

- Make sure that you have discarded all cigarettes and cigarette lighters. Smokers have a propensity to keep a cigarette around the house, in the car, or at work, just in case.

- Invest some of your newly saved cigarette money in a new perfume or cologne. When you stop smoking, your body will smell entirely different.

- Tell everyone you know that you have quit smoking.

Stop Smoking Wellness Rx for Withdrawal Week

In addition to your seven Wellness Rx promises, this week promise to do the following:

- Recite the Serenity Prayer each morning.
- Practice random acts of kindness.
- Practice the breathing techniques and easy yoga postures described in Chapter Seven.
- Make your environment smoke-free.
- Change your behavior to discourage smoke-related thoughts.

  I hereby vow on my honor and integrity to fulfill these promises.

  _____

  (your signature and today's date)

THE REINFORCEMENT WEEK

Turn your face to the sun and the shadows fall behind you.
—Maori proverb

Congratulations on Not Smoking!

You have come to the third stage of the De-addiction Process. You have already successfully completed the declaration and withdrawal stages, and you are about to become one of the tens of millions of ex-smokers who just simply stopped forever. Smoking no longer needs to be a part of your life.

The refill of the Stop Smoking Wellness Rx for this week consists of the same twelve promises you followed last week but deepens the spiritual basis of your commitment to never smoke again. Review your twelve promises involving the following:

1. The Serenity Prayer
2. Meditation
3. Limit alcohol and caffeine
4. Energy nutrition
5. Exercise
6. The Golden Rule
7. Unconditional love
8. Be happy, not right
9. Random acts of kindness
10. Environmental change
11. Behavioral change
12. Yoga and breathing

Play a Higher Role

To further your mental detachment from your former addiction, you may find it helpful to just regard yourself as an actor or an actress playing a role on the stage. For this next week, you'll be reciting the same lines and acting the same way, constantly aware of not forgetting your lines and your cues. Thus, you'll observe yourself carrying out the same twelve promises each day of the performance, following the same routine you have committed to memory. Imagine ancient curtains pulling apart in your mind. Let the grand play open. Your life becomes a stage and you are the star.

Reinforcement

The De-addiction Process is very much like a time-management problem until you are free of nicotine forever. You just need something else to do when you are experiencing feelings or engaged in activities that made you reach for a cigarette less than three weeks ago. In the life of a smoker each act and each feeling is connected to a corresponding smoking act. Think about the activities you formerly did while smoking. The typical smoker associates smoking with the following activities:

Activities Linked to Smoking	Feelings Linked to Smoking
• waking up——smoking	• boredom——smoking
• bathroom——smoking	• excitement——smoking
• showering——smoking	• loneliness——smoking
• shaving——smoking	• anger——smoking
• applying makeup——smoking	• anxiety——smoking
• coffee——smoking	• depression——smoking
• eating——smoking	• disappointment——smoking
• working——smoking	• frustration——smoking
• sex——smoking	• worry——smoking
• driving——smoking	• fear——smoking

Depend on Your Higher Connections

You may feel this week that something is missing, some connection just isn't being made. That is because the activities you engaged in and the feelings you experienced were connected to the act of smoking, whether you were conscious of this connection or not. It was just like a long linked chain of events and feelings that were linked up with your puffing madly away. Now there are gaps in the chain as you have become free again. During the last two weeks you have been creating soulful ways of filling in those gaps. *Higher connections,* one might say. Just as all the associations between smoking and acts and feelings were created, they were crumbled. This is the process you have been engaged in for the last two weeks. Be increasingly aware now of the "health-full," "soul-full" associations you have created in place of the deadly addiction.

The connections remind me of a bicycle chain in which each link requires a corresponding sprocket on the gear to fit into. The entire mechanism gets jammed if there is a missing linkup. The bike then breaks down. Smokers' brains require corresponding linkups between certain activities and nicotine to function comfortably too. Or they feel they will break down.

The bicycle chain works well only with each link engaging neatly with the sprockets on the gear. You fashioned your life with cigarettes that way too. Even though smoking is irrelevant to you, there still will be times when you feel you are indeed missing a link or two. The following steps will allow you to make thoughtful higher substitutions for the gaps whenever you experience a painful confrontation with a moment that previously called for a cigarette.

Higher Substitutions

1. Remind yourself that the acute craving will be gone within twenty seconds.
2. Take three slow, deep breaths while curling your toes. Silently say to yourself, with each breath: "I AM NO LONGER A SMOKER!"
3. Deepen your spiritual commitment by remembering that you have said yes to those who love you, to those you love, and to life itself.

When you say yes to God, God says yes, yes, yes a million times to you. This unquestionable faith is your greatest source of freedom from your former addiction.

TERMINATION

The greatest human quest is to know what one must do in order to become a human being.
—Immanuel Kant

By all visible measures, you are no longer a smoker. You may therefore be questioning whether you even need to complete this last week of De-addiction Process. It depends. If you slipped and smoked *even one time* during the last week, it is absolutely **crucial** that you complete this last week. Remember that you are *healing* the inner source of your addiction, and healing is a process, not an event.

Even if you followed the promises exactly, you will likely still feel the need for ongoing support and healing. Quiet your thoughts using the meditation technique you are now familiar with and then, in that stillness and peace, ask yourself with all of your heart and soul if you are truly free of your addiction. If the answer from your heart and soul is "I am no longer a smoker," you may skip this last week of the program.

For most of you, this will be the crucial step in driving the final wedge between you and your former addiction. Consider this your grand finale. By the end of this week you will have formed new mental blueprints that will etch themselves more deeply into your mind over time. These are the subtle pathways of energy that determine your health destiny. You created these blueprints. Your health destiny is in your hands.

The Declaration Week

Day 1	Day 2	Day 3	Day 4	Day 5	Day 6	Day 7
1. Addiction	1. Addiction	1. Addiction	1. Addiction	1. Addiction	1. Addiction	1. Addiction
2. Nutrition	2. Nutrition	2. Nutrition	2. Nutrition	2. Nutrition	2. Nutrition	2. Nutrition
3. Exercise	3. Exercise	3. Exercise	3. Exercise	3. Exercise	3. Exercise	3. Exercise
4. Lovingness	4. Lovingness	4. Lovingness	4. Lovingness	4. Lovingness	4. Lovingness	4. Lovingness
5. Golden Rule	5. Golden Rule	5. Golden Rule	5. Golden Rule	5. Golden Rule	5. Golden Rule	5. Golden Rule
6. Meditation	6. Meditation	6. Meditation	6. Meditation	6. Meditation	6. Meditation	6. Meditation
7. Happy, Not Right	7. Happy, Not Right	7. Happy, Not Right	7. Happy, Not Right	7. Happy, Not Right	7. Happy, Not Right	7. Happy, Not Right
8. Serenity Prayer	8. Serenity Prayer	8. Serenity Prayer	8. Serenity Prayer	8. Serenity Prayer	8. Serenity Prayer	8. Continue Promises
9. Butt Jar	9. Butt Jar	9. Butt Jar	9. Butt Jar	9. Butt Jar	9. Butt Jar	9. Throw Away Cigarettes
10. Smoke Outside	10. Smoke Outside	10. Smoke Outside	10. Smoke Outside	10. Smoke Outside	10. Smoke Outside	10. Last Cigarette By Midnight
11. Cut Down	11. Cut Down	11. Cut Down	11. Cut Down	11. Cut Down	11. Cut Down	

The Withdrawal Week

Day 1	Day 2	Day 3	Day 4	Day 5	Day 6	Day 7
1. Addiction	1.	1.	1.	1.	1.	1.
2. Nutrition	2.	2.	2.	2.	2.	2.
3. Exercise	3.	3.	3.	3.	3.	3.
4. Lovingness	4.	4.	4.	4.	4.	4.
5. Golden Rule	5.	5.	5.	5.	5.	5.
6. Meditation	6.	6.	6.	6.	6.	6.
7. Happy, Not Right	7.	7.	7.	7.	7.	7.
8. Serenity Prayer	8.	8.	8.	8.	8.	8.
9. Act of Kindness	9.	9.	9.	9.	9.	9.
10. Breathe/Yoga	10.	10.	10.	10.	10.	10.
11. Environment	11.	11.	11.	11.	11.	11.
12. Behavior	12.	12.	12.	12.	12.	12.

The Reinforcement Week

Day 1	Day 2	Day 3	Day 4	Day 5	Day 6	Day 7
1. Addiction	1.	1.	1.	1.	1.	1.
2. Nutrition	2.	2.	2.	2.	2.	2.
3. Exercise	3.	3.	3.	3.	3.	3.
4. Lovingness	4.	4.	4.	4.	4.	4.
5. Golden Rule	5.	5.	5.	5.	5.	5.
6. Meditation	6.	6.	6.	6.	6.	6.
7. Happy, Not Right	7.	7.	7.	7.	7.	7.
8. Serenity Prayer	8.	8.	8.	8.	8.	8.
9. Act of Kindness	9.	9.	9.	9.	9.	9.
10. Breathe/Yoga	10.	10.	10.	10.	10.	10.
11. Environment	11.	11.	11.	11.	11.	11.
12. Behavior	12.	12.	12.	12.	12.	12.

15

SAY GOODBYE TO

BACK PAIN

If you have back pain, you are among the nearly 95 percent of Americans who report they suffer from an aching back. Back pain is the second leading reason for office visits to physicians and the number one reason for sick leave from work. In 1992 Americans spent about 30 billion dollars looking for some relief from their pain. Billions are spent annually on CAT scans, x-rays, and imaging procedures that may or may not reveal the cause of pain, and subsequent billions are spent on drastic surgical procedures that may not even target the source of the pain. Most of these patients will leave the operating room to eventually seek nonsurgical interventions to address the recurring pain.

Most patients I see in my office for back pain share a common misperception about their discomfort. Although probably less than 5 percent of back pain is caused by a structural abnormality of the spine, most patients tell me things like: "I think I have a slipped disk" or "I think I pinched a nerve." The great majority of backaches are not related to problems in the vertebrae, disks, or spine. Backaches usually originate in the soft tissue, muscles, nerves, and tendons surrounding the spine and lower-back region.

TOO MUCH REST CAN HURT

A general misunderstanding about backache and its proper treatment has been shared by physicians. For years, the standard treatments for back pain have been either surgery or prolonged bed rest. But recent studies indicate that a lengthy period of bed rest actually exacerbates lower-back pain by restricting the blood flow to the back region and contributing to muscle weakness in the legs and hips. Not long ago it was routine for doctors to recommend two weeks in bed for back pain. Numerous studies, however, are now finding that, in fact, gentle stretching and moderate exercise are the best medicine for back pain. Stretching and exercise have even provided permanent relief for longtime sufferers of back pain, including those with the sharp, burning pain of sciatica.

What about relief from back pain related to a serious underlying systemic disease, such as cancer or spinal infection? In fact, very few backaches result from these causes. You may be surprised to hear also that only a very small percentage of back pain can be tied to a recent fall, injury, or physical strain. While herniated disks, tumors, osteoarthritis, injuries, and other illnesses should always be carefully and systematically ruled out by a skilled physician, research is now showing that the majority of back pain is almost always related to emotional or mental stress. Consequently, most backaches can be remedied without expensive surgeries. The Wellness Rx for Backache presents a comprehensive strategy for alleviating not only back pain but the *source* of that pain, quickly and permanently.

When I say that backache results from mental or emotional stress, I do not mean that physical injuries or accidents do not play a part. I merely mean that for the average person with back pain—nine out of every ten Americans with backache—the pain is not a result of recent or past injury but a direct response to stress. Most back pain is in the soft tissues of the back, not in the bones. Remember that every belief, attitude, anger, worry, fear, or anxiety that you have in your mind is broadcasted out to every cell in your body. The cells that make up the ligaments and muscles of your lower back tend to be a clearinghouse for those harmful messages. If given the opportunity, those destructive responses to stress, communicated to all of the cells in your body, will imbed themselves deeply in the muscle tissues surrounding the lower back. The message received by the hip, back, and buttocks muscles causes them to tense up, tighten, and strain. This muscle action is what results in spasm and backache.

MENTAL SURGERY

When you become aware that the pain in your back is not structural, that is, not "in the bones," then it becomes clear that any treatment strategy that seeks to provide permanent relief must address the true source of the ache. Unless you have a history of cancer or you have recently been in a physical accident, it is almost certain that your back pain is related to emotional or mental stress. In that case, do not have surgery on your back.

What you need to do instead is perform "mental surgery" on your responses and reactions to stressful experiences. Mental surgery means uprooting harmful, illness-inviting beliefs and attitudes and replacing them with wellness-provoking ones, the very same process I have been describing throughout this book. It is necessary to cultivate new mental blueprints that do not include in their template any room for backache. Mental surgery for backache entails that you first become aware that while your pain may be excruciatingly physical, the source of that pain is rooted in your mind and soul.

Clearly, surgical intervention has provided only minimal relief for backache at best, and in many cases has actually made the pain worse. It is time to acknowledge not only the mental and emotional underpinnings of back pain but strategies for lasting relief, ones that address the pain at the level of mind and soul.

Back Tracks

Take a step backward. Create a mental image of the anatomy and physiology of the back so that you can properly conceptualize your back pain as essentially stress-related. The back is a column of bones called vertebrae. Separating the vertebrae are disks, which are like firm, gelatinous cushions. Muscles, cartilage, ligaments, and tendons hold the back bones in place and receive nourishment from blood vessels, arteries, veins, capillaries, and a lymphatic drainage system.

Passing through the vertebrae like liquid through a straw is the spinal cord, with a complex system of nerves that extend throughout the entire body. The spinal cord is like a major interstate highway, and the spinal nerves are responsible for coordinating the traffic of trillions and trillions of messages traveling from and to the brain from every part of the body. A disruption in any one of the supporting structures of the spine can lead to pain that grips the entire back.

Pain in the back can be caused by imbalances in the energy of other parts of the body as well. Difficulty in the gallbladder, prostate gland, uterus, kidneys, and even the heart can incite the back to ache if that happens to be your physical point of least resistance—the Achilles heel, as it were.

Given what you already know about how much damage cigarette smoking does to the energy system of the body, it may not surprise you that smoking inflames an already tender back. Smoking chokes the flow of blood, oxygen, and energy in the body. When energy in the back muscles is already constricted as a response to emotional or mental stress, the blood flow to those tissues is already below normal and may just be made worse by smoking.

At a more subtle level, the spine is the center of your body's energy system. Practitioners of yoga speak of the "subtle spine" not only as the highway along which information and impulses to and from your brain are transmitted but also the central pathway of energy throughout your body, mind, and soul. The spine is a channel of life energy, or *prana*. Life energy is drawn into the body through the breath and concentrated in the spine. Since smoking alters normal breathing, obstructing the flow of life energy, it also thwarts the flow of energy in your spine. So from the perspective of the "subtle spine," it is not difficult to see how smoking can exacerbate back pain.

CREATING PERMANENT RELIEF

The Wellness Rx for Backache is based on the understanding of the body as a total energy system. Surgery that removes a herniated disk, chiropractic care that temporarily "adjusts" the spine, aspirin or muscle relaxants that temporarily numb the pain can be appropriate treatments for backache. But they are only temporary treatments. The Wellness Rx for Backache will help you create permanent relief by restoring the balance of energy that has been upset and caused the backache in the first place. This Rx moves the focus away from your physical pain, as excruciating as it may be, and targets the beliefs, attitudes, and emotions that underlie the pain. When you grasp the fact that the origins of your pain are largely manufactured in your mind, then permanent relief is already beginning to take over.

TWELVE IMPORTANT STEPS TO FOLLOW

The Rx for healing backache builds upon the basic Wellness Rx laid out in Chapter Three. *In addition* to the promises you are making regarding nutrition, exercise, lovingness, meditation, happiness, and ethics, the guidelines listed here must be followed to promote permanent relief from backache.

- Sleep on a mattress or surface that is extra firm. Slipping a board under your mattress will solve the problems of a slouchy bed. Use a small, soft pillow, or no pillow at all. You may find it helpful to place a pillow beneath your knees when you sleep on your back. This will release the pressure on your lower back as well as prevent you from falling into an awkward sleeping position that may strain your back.

- Take a long, hot bath or Jacuzzi every day for seven days. A hot shower will do if a bathtub is unavailable, concentrating the hot water on your lower back.

- In addition to the dietary guidelines agreed to in the basic Wellness Rx, as a backache sufferer you need to avoid constipation. Stay within the top five rungs of the Food Energy Ladder. Fresh fruits and uncooked vegetables help regulate the digestive and elimination processes. A Dulcolax® suppository or a Fleets® disposable enema can be helpful. In most cases, lots of roughage and exercise will be sufficient.

- Use anti-inflammatory medicine as needed. Ibuprofen, Acetomenophen or aspirin used in correct amounts every six to eight hours are very helpful. Many of these medicines are irritative to the stomach and should be switched or stopped if there is a problem.

- Take two general therapeutic strength multivitamin and mineral tablets and 2000 to 3000 mg of vitamin C daily.

- Get a massage. The professional touch of a masseur or masseuse or a physical therapist helps to restore balance to the body's energy system, particularly in the back. If professional massage is unavailable, a relative or friend can easily follow illustrated directions in any of a number of good books on massage. A massage every 2 or 3 days while your back is aching would be ideal.

- Choose light exercises and do them for a total of twenty minutes daily, every day this week. Walking, jogging, bicycling, or swimming will help loosen the muscles in the back and keep the muscles flexible. Contrary to conventional wisdom, exercise will increase your strength and decrease your pain.

- Gentle stretching exercises, twice daily, will help release tension in the back muscles and encourage strength and flexibility, which help prevent backache. Follow the easy yoga routine detailed in Chapter Seven, after you get out of bed in the morning and before you go to bed in the evening.

- To help relieve pressure on the hips and back, make simple adjustments in where you carry your wallet or purse. Men should not carry their wallet in the back pocket, and women should avoid carrying purses over their shoulders. And women who experience backache definitely must not wear high heels.

- Correct posture, while standing and sitting, is crucial. Posture is often a reflection of attitude. Motivated, energetic people tend to carry their shoulders back, chin tilted slightly upward, the spine straightened toward the sky. Depressed and tired people tend to slouch their shoulders, drop their chin toward the ground, and hunch their spine forward. Changes in posture can inspire changes in attitude and vice versa.

- A positive, healthful environment is important. Where weather permits, open the windows for fresh air; draw back the curtains to let in fresh light. Peaceful music can be uplifting and relaxing.

- Finally, this Rx calls for moderate rest but *not* immobility. If possible, take a short vacation, and always take an hour for personal retreat and relaxation during the day. While resting, unplug the phone, read an inspiring or humorous book, and enjoy the solitude. The ideal thing to do is to get away from whatever you would normally do for a day. Become so totally removed from the ordinary that nothing would trigger a stressful response. You can even go skiing!

The Emotional Anatomy of Back Pain

The practical guidelines for relieving backache are fairly straightforward and certainly do not require that you go too far out of your way to comply. Interestingly enough, however, I have seen many patients, including members of my family, fail to adopt the recommendations. Even after following the guidelines and having no back pain for a full week, my own mother, brother, and daughter each abandoned the Rx. Why were they unwilling to continue the practices proven to provide relief from their pain even after experiencing an entire week free of pain?

Permanent relief from back pain requests its sufferers to release the tension in their back muscles, but even more important, to let go of the thoughts, beliefs, and emotions underlying the physical tension. I am convinced that this is the major obstacle facing back-pain sufferers. If we know we can live without back pain, why do we then choose not to follow the practices that relieve the pain? Because we're not sure that we can learn to live without all of the feelings, thoughts, emotions, and attitudes that are the cement holding our backache in place. Letting go of these mental blueprints, years in the making, is not an easy task. But it can be done, and the rewards are forever.

CASE HISTORY—LETTING GO OF SELF-DOUBT AND BLAME

To illustrate just how difficult it is to release the beliefs and feelings underlying pain, even when doing so would free you of the pain, let me share the story of a woman, fifty-two years of age, who came to me with a backache so severe she could barely sit. When Patricia walked into my office, I immediately felt the impulse to approach her and pull her shoulders back. Her shoulders were so hunched forward that her entire chest seemed to sink like a canyon. Her body language sent out a message of tremendous sorrow, and her shoulders seemed to collapse around whatever she was carrying on her chest, as if to protect her.

Patricia stated that she had had lower-back pain on and off for the last ten years. She described the pain as barely tolerable by day, excruciating by night. She also described occasional pain radiating to her left calf and her left sole, as well as some numbness and tingling in that area. My physical examination was normal, and x-rays revealed mild degenerative disease of her third and fourth lumbar disks and a slight left-sided scoliosis. After ruling out a herniated disk, tumor, or other systemic illness, I determined that she had acute and chronic lumbosacral muscle sprain, with mild radiculitis and osteoarthritis, none of which required surgical intervention.

Together Patricia and I mapped out a Wellness Rx for her backache based on the guidelines above. After going through each of the components, I asked Patricia if she thought she could agree to follow the Wellness Rx.

"Well, basically it just means I have to be good to my back and myself for a week, right?"

"Exactly. But tell me, are you usually not good to your back or yourself?"

Patricia hesitated and shrugged her shoulders even higher. "I know that I carry a lot of emotions around with me. There's nowhere to put them, so I keep them inside. But I accept that."

I wondered what she was accepting. "Perhaps when you come back next week, if you wish, we might talk about those emotions and how they might be contributing to your back pain." We agreed to meet in seven days, after she had followed the Wellness Rx for one week. When she returned to my office, her posture was slightly better, but she seemed fairly down. Apparently she had had no difficulty following the Rx and reported that after the second day her backache had nearly disappeared. She continued to follow the guidelines precisely and was free of pain until the sixth day. On the sixth day she did not meditate and ate a plate of pork roast at a friend's dinner party. That night she had awful diarrhea, and the pain in her lower back returned. The pain was so bad the next day, she stated that she nearly canceled her appointment with me because getting in and out of her car was now nearly impossible.

Patricia was willing to start again, but it was clear that the backache was reflecting an underlying emotional disruption that still needed to be addressed. I prescribed a mild anti-inflammatory medication and suggested that she restart her Wellness Rx. I asked her if she felt good during the first few days without pain. "Yes, but I just felt so selfish taking all that time out for myself—the meditation, stretching, hot baths, that stuff. You know my son has some behavioral and learning problems, and I spend a lot of time working with him. It was hard for me to find the time to do all of those things for me last week."

As we talked about her son, who was also under my care, it became clear to both of us that the pain in Patricia's back was actually a cry from her soul for more attention, more love and forgiveness. She admitted that she blamed herself for some of her son's learning difficulties and was deeply committed to helping him in every way she possibly could. She also admitted that she didn't feel like she could ever do enough. Patricia agreed to follow the Wellness Rx and the specific steps to relieve backache for another week, this time concentrating on loving *herself* unconditionally. When she stood to leave my office after our appointment, her shoulders seemed a bit more relaxed. Patricia scheduled a follow-up for one week later.

But Patricia did not come back. I didn't see her again for four months, when she came in for her son's school physical. While I checked her son's tonsils I asked her how her back was feeling. She reported that her pain was still present most of the time, but that she was learning to live with it. I extended her an open invitation for another consultation, which she has yet to follow through on.

Patricia experienced five days without back pain. She learned how to let go of the pain. But then she stopped. She wasn't willing or ready to learn how to let go of the deep feelings of self-doubt and blame that dwell beneath the surface of her pain, deeper than the muscles and tissues of her back. I still don't know enough about Patricia's history to know why she was not ready to address her beliefs and feelings. But I have seen this pattern so consistently to believe that back pain results from some of our most difficult emotions. Is it possible that we think accessing these emotions will somehow be more painful than the back pain itself? Is that why people choose to live with the pain instead of let it go? Are people reluctant to pursue the path to freedom from back pain because it requires confronting painful or difficult thoughts, forgiving themselves, or surrendering to a Higher Power?

For many, perhaps, temporary relief from back pain is enough—until the next bout of anger, worry, desire, or frustration occurs. But I'd like you to believe that you can have more. Taking control of your back pain forever requires that you take control of the burdensome beliefs and feelings that have made a home out of the tension and strain in your back. Follow the Wellness Rx with the guidelines for relieving backache permanently and you will make your back, and your entire body, a home for peace and joy instead.

BACKACHE WELLNESS TREATMENT PROGRAM

An effective failure. That's what this backache treatment plan is. Sounds like an oxymoron, doesn't it? Let me explain: it is so simple and so effective that 95% of my patients have refused the treatment because it helps so much!

In a consecutive series of fifty backache patients, including my mother, my brother, my wife, my nephew and myself, forty-five patients declined the prescription or stopped compliance with it by the fourth or fifth day. The only patients who were helped were my mother, my brother, my wife, my nephew and myself; this chapter is ultimately their story and a true testimony to the healing power of both love and forgiveness.

This section describes some of the patient—failures and all of the patient—successes, to help backache sufferers understand the overall nature of the problem, beginning with its psychopathophysiology. Because, would you believe that the last thing a typical backache sufferer is actually prepared for, is for the backache to go away? It's true.

What is also absolutely true is that the vast majority of backaches begin with a physical cause (a twisting motion, a fall, lifting too heavy an object or lifting it incorrectly, a car or work related-accident). Basically, the injury causes the paraspinous muscles on either side of the spine to go into spasm causing pain, causing more spasm, causing more pain, causing more spasm. A vicious cycle ensues: like a ball rolling downhill that will continue to roll and pick up speed because of the force of gravity, the injured muscles will continue to spasm and experience an increased intensity until the driving force behind it has dissipated.

What is the driving force? Initially it's pain. Then it's the muscle spasm. Subsequently, however, it's much much more and this is from where the vast majority of the people making up the legions of backache sufferers arise. The subsequent driving force is basically fear and anger. And anxiety and depression. Also memory of past experience. Secondary gain, too, and excuses from obligations.

The common denominator among all the patients was uttering the phrase: "Doctor, I would do anything to get better."

The common denominator among those who did not get better was deciding immediately or within five days that it was just *"too much of a bother"* to follow their promises—to meditate, to exercise, to stretch, to eat appropriately, to love someone unconditionally, or to follow the golden rule.

THE EX-SUFFERER'S CREED

We all understand your pain because we have suffered with backache too. Until it was enough. We all resisted surrendering to a Higher Power and letting go of hurt, resentment, anger and fear. Then we declared that the suffering was enough and we became well.

You too can be cured of your backache. The beginning of your power occurs with awareness—awareness of stored up anger, resentment, sorrow and hurt in your mind. Suppressed emotions are enormous boulders that you carry on your back. The healing Force easily removes the boulders from your back and allows suffering to end.

Now is the time to declare total surrender and unconditional amnesty and forgiveness (for yourself and others). Sign the Wellness Rx (on page 108) and add the new ingredients covered in this chapter.

16
ANGELS OF ENERGY

Almost all the major medical traditions outside of Western medicine are grounded in the unifying concept of life energy. Even though all those other medical systems are very specific to their own country and culture, it is amazing that they share in common a basic understanding of energy as vitality, a life force. Hindus call this life energy *prana,* a life force or vitality that sustains each human body as well as the universe. In Chinese medicine and culture, this life force is *chi,* the vital energy that flows through every human and living thing in the universe. Ancient Chinese physicians taught and practiced "energy medicine," therapies developed to balance disruptions of energy and to stimulate the life force in the patient. The Wellness Rx combines the best that modern Western medicine offers with the Eastern awareness that within every human body is a vital life force.

A GLORIOUS COMPOSITION

Like the musical score to an enchanting symphony, our lives and the universe we inhabit are knit together by a great underlying tone, a universal chord. Each of us is an expression of a heavenly rhythm, moving through our daily lives in tune with the melody of a spellbinding music. Dr. Larry Dossey calls it a "Great Tone" and suggests calm to hear the energy of the music flowing gently throughout our body. I perceive it as a magnificent resonance and marvel at how very much different the body looks and feels from this perspective—not an unfeeling machine, but a glorious composition of silent music played in solitude.

For decades, we have been spiritually shipwrecked. This is the source of much of our illness and suffering. We have forgotten that we are small waves that are part of a larger ocean. Thinking of ourselves only as individual waves has separated us from the boundless universal sea of energy. To find a way back to the infinite ocean of peace and wellness, we need to enhance the flow of the body's life energy. To attune our minds once again to the "Great Resonance," we need to "turn up the volume" of our homeostasis and tune into the Healing Force that flows within us. We have become like radios stuck in between two frequencies, overwhelmed by static and dissonance. The Wellness Rx will stir up the energy within you that is necessary to put yourself back in perfect tune.

Life, after all, is a human symphony as well as a divine comedy. Living through it may not be comfortable or seem comical at times, but live through it we must, as we search for meaning. The process of life itself, the joys and the ordeals, is healing. When we are attuned to the Healing Force we no longer think of ourselves as isolated waves, limited to this body, this flesh, this face we see in the mirror. We see ourselves instead as part of a wonderful sea of souls whose joys are far superior to those we experience as our limited individual selves. This same feeling is expressed by the poet William Blake and deserves quoting once more:

> *To see a World in a grain of sand*
> *And a Heaven in a wild flower,*
> *Hold Infinity in the palm of your hand,*
> *And Eternity in an hour.*

To the extent that you can see a world in a grain of sand, to the extent that you can see the essence of all life in one person, you can experience this joy. From this awareness, the experience of connectedness with the whole universe, no illness can destroy your balance. Blake's words echo those of an enchanting Hindu poem: "When one sees Eternity in things that pass away and Infinity in finite things, then one has pure knowledge." And eternity in an hour. Pure knowledge, perfect expression of inner wisdom, an understanding of the invisible thread that weaves our tiny lives into the vast blanket of this universe—this is the foundation upon which wellness emerges.

BENEATH A HALO OF HEALTH

In the first chapters of this book we explored the habits of mind, body, and soul that help you enhance the flow of your body's Healing Force. Despite any illness or disease, under the toughest adversities, your Healing Force lies kindled quietly within your soul, just waiting to be recharged. The strategies and stories described in this book help to fan that flame, to illuminate your soul, calm the restless waves of your mind, and set you sailing once again on the sea of energy from which you were born.

An Indian sage once told his students: "God made us angels of energy, encased in solids—currents of life dazzling through a material bulb of flesh. But through concentration on the frailties and fragility of the body bulb, we have forgotten how to feel the immortal, indestructible properties of the eternal life energy within the mutable flesh."* This book is directed toward enabling you to recharge that life energy, to live and be well, just like an angel of energy.

The next part of this chapter will help you understand how and why this vital source within us has been dimmed, why our angel's wings have lost their energy, burdened by stress, illness, and disease. Before reading on, let your mind linger quietly on the following affirmation, designed to begin the process of lifting the burden from the wings of wellness that were meant to protect you from illness. Affirmations are meaningful statements heard at the level of the soul. They are soulful prayers with a purpose and a promise. Try not to analyze, because your conscious mind will not understand. Indulge your imagination instead. For now, be content to be curious, but not inquisitive.

EXERCISE FOR RECHARGING LIFE ENERGY

Imagine that the words below are a beautiful hymn or spiritual song. Read the affirmation, silently at first, listening to the rhythm of the words and the melody they make in your mind.

Repeat the affirmation silently three times. Then whisper the words softly to yourself, three times, as if you were telling yourself a sacred secret.

Repeat the affirmation again, this time speaking at the level of your regular speaking voice. Listen to the sound the words make; hear the melody in the sentences as you speak them, slowly, with intent, three times.

Repeat the affirmation again, returning to a whisper, quietly speaking to yourself. Finally, silently again repeat the affirmation. After you complete this process, sit quietly for a moment with your eyes closed and be aware of the peace and quiet that surrounds you.

This is the music of the soul.

---

*Paramahansa Yogananda, *Where There Is Light* (Los Angeles: Self Realization Fellowship, 1988)

I am part of a glorious composition.
Divine music surrounds me
and casts its healing light
in every cell of my body.
I live my life in harmony with
the Song of my Soul.

SHIFTING VISIONS

This book helps establish the principles of a new paradigm for Soulful Medicine. Most important, its emphasis is on teaching you the practical habits and attitudes that will cultivate radiant energy and passionate, vital, *soulful* health.

Science lost its soul in the seventeenth century, when the world of science exploded and opened up entirely new ways of thinking about the world and the human being's place in it. Ironically, this historical era was known as the Enlightenment.

The most prominent Enlightenment philosopher, René Descartes, decreed that the world of knowable objects and observations that constituted science and the unmeasurable world of the mind and soul were absolutely discrete and different entities. Mankind was for the first time declared completely separate from nature.

As a result of the divided universe envisioned by Descartes, science recoiled from theology and philosophy and restricted its inquiry solely to what could be measured and governed by logic and reason. *Soulful Medicine begins by mending this artificial separation.*

Imagination Is the Source of All Creativity

It is precisely because science now operates only in the realm of that which can be quantified and measured that many modern physicians are so uncomfortable dealing with the terrain of the soul—that space or substance that eludes definition and is beyond measure. Because of its seemingly remote quality, the soul bumps up against the materialistic foundations of modern medicine.

Although the language of the soul defies "rational" explanation and measurement, what we do not know may be just as important as what we do know, in this age of overwhelming stress. Yet in the oft-turned pages of all of my medical textbooks, of the *Physician's Desk Reference*, no entry on the essential healing quality of the soul exists. And yet the soul expresses itself in all forms of illness, just as it is the inspiration underlying all methods of healing. Just because the *PDR* cannot define it does not mean its presence is not revealed in millions of ways everyday. Imagination itself is the light of the soul. A contemporary philosopher of science explains the nature of the puzzle perfectly: "Definition is an intellectual enterprise. . . . The soul prefers to imagine."[*]

Imagination, indeed, has been the source of many celebrated medical innovations. Before he could develop a vaccine for polio, Jonas Salk had to imagine its possibility. Fleming's discovery of penicillin must have been fueled by his imagination. How else could he think that a mold growing on bread could wipe out any number of germs in the body? Where was the idea born, if not in the imagination, that genes could be spliced to artificially produce insulin? Whether we attribute it to genius or determination or a combination of both, imagination is always present in the work of great physicians. Imagination, indeed, is the root of all creativity. If we are to create wellness, we must learn to be as imaginative as often as we are scientific.

Medicine Under the Microscope

One of the characteristic attributes of so-called scientific medical practice is its objectivity. Webster's Dictionary defines *objective* as "independent of mind." By definition, then, objective medical science exists outside of subjective feeling or prejudice. In practice, however, scientific medicine *is* prejudiced, with a strong bias against the mind and a total exclusion of the soul. No other myth has more profoundly shaped modern medicine than the myth of the divided body, mind, and soul.

Every medical student inherits this Enlightenment period viewpoint as his or her conceptual tool to organize, diagnose, and treat the physical body. The practices of modern medicine are organized around a particular way of seeing the human being and a particular way of making sense out of the trillions of processes occurring in the body at any given second. But this way of seeing, this Cartesian viewpoint, is merely a subjective interpretation and opinion. The scientific traditional medical viewpoint is not a figurative window peering out onto the world, a transparent veil that neither distorts nor disturbs "reality." It is like a lens, shaped and curved,

---

[*]Thomas Moore, *Care of the Soul* (New York: Harper Collins, 1992), xi.

filtering an image of the world through its own prejudiced contours and perspective.

The practice of medicine is, at a very fundamental level, the practice of a set of culturally determined beliefs about the human body and disease. Diagnosis is the process of interpreting an array of information including physical symptoms and patient history within the framework provided by these sets of beliefs. Medical diagnosis is the interplay between intellect and imagination, a conversation between the observed and the anticipated. Chinese, Russian, Indian, African and American physicians see the same patient in a different way. Even French and American physicians see the same patient in a different way!

Modern medicine, supposedly objective and based in material and observable truths, rests upon a bias toward mechanics and biology. As the most skilled and compassionate physicians defend this bias as necessary to ensure the finest and most technically advanced patient treatment, they have a hard time recognizing the extent to which this priority limits not only their view of the body and disease but most important the resources available to assist in the healing process—those belonging to patients themselves.

In his book *Planet Medicine*, anthropologist Richard Grossinger describes ancient and present systems of healing around the world, demonstrating that there are as many ways of thinking about and treating human disease as there are cultures. "In any culture, the medical establishment 'establishes' customs of belief and treatment as the political establishment evolves laws and an economic establishment determines the basis of exchange."* Clearly, part of what binds a culture together are the definitions of life's experiences—the meanings attributed to birth, sickness, God, family, sex, food, age, death—shared by members of that culture.

Learning to practice medicine involves learning to put *into* practice a whole set of beliefs, attitudes, and assumptions about the human body, disease, and scientific knowledge. These practices and meanings are culturally specific; that is, they differ according to particular cultural and historical contexts.

Difference, however, does not mean deficient. The problem of our medical system—much like our economic and political systems—is that its practitioners and advocates tend to treat different, or alternative, health-

---

*Richard Grossinger, *Planet Medicine: From Stone Age Shamanism to Post-industrial Medicine*, 5th ed. (Berkeley, CA: North Atlantic Books, 1990), 27.

care practices within our own and other cultures as inferior to the Western medical standard. Orthodox Western medicine typically sees itself as the sole or superior means of addressing disease. In a limited sense, this is true. The technical power of modern European and American medicine is impressive and possibly the most effective apparatus for accomplishing what this medical establishment is geared toward: *disease repair.*

But then again, not all medical systems are organized around repairing disease once it is present in the body. Many systems of healing emphasize preventive measures undertaken *before* the onset of disease, while many others approach illness from an entirely spiritual standpoint. The fact is that those of us who live in the United States live in a "quick-fix" society, preferring superficial treatments over those that require even minor changes in our lifestyle, beliefs, and attitudes, and delaying such change until it is absolutely imperative. For this, our high-tech, acute-crisis-oriented medical system serves us well.

But high-tech, crisis-oriented care does not address the underlying factors keeping us from being well. Indeed, in an astonishingly high number of cases, orthodox treatments actually cause or worsen our injuries and are responsible for thousands of patient deaths a year. Medical malpractice alone is responsible for 45,000 deaths annually and is the major cause of accidental injury and death. A recent Rand Corporation study revealed that one-fourth of all surgery performed in this country's hospitals—totaling $132 billion—is unnecessary.

In our lifetimes, very few of us will actually suffer the traumatic injuries and critical conditions that conventional medicine is so expertly equipped to treat; what we need, and what the disease-repair system does not provide, is satisfactory care for the chronic conditions like headache, insomnia, arthritis, back trouble, anxiety, fatigue, hypertension, and colitis that cloud our daily lives.

Limitations of the Medical Model

Clearly, the cultural framework within which orthodox medicine has emerged has made possible medical innovations far too numerous to count, many of which are now taken for granted, including CAT scans, magnetic resonance imagining, organ transplantation, and genetic engineering. But the cultural definitions of human health and illness inherited from the Enlightenment have also hindered our pursuit of wellness. Even the most humanitarian physicians are constrained by the cultural values and "taboos" that define their professional practice.

THE GREAT TABOO OF MODERN MEDICINE

One of the most stubborn taboos in Western medicine is any reference to the soul. Modern physicians are trained minimally if at all in the art of deep human interaction. What they basically learn is how to allay fear and anxiety in the patient by appearing calm and competent at all times.

In the last several years, an entirely new science has developed called psychoneuroimmunology. The pursuit of this scientific inquiry has increased our understanding of the relationship between the mind and body and the ways that feelings and emotions influence health and disease. Groundbreaking research has demonstrated that the mind literally exists in every cell of the body. Every thought, every attitude, every inkling of an idea, expresses itself in every cell of our body through a chemical communications network that scientists knew very little about until just recently.

The practices described in this book deepen and broaden what has come to be known as mind/body medicine. In this book I introduce readers to a medicine for the soul. This soul-filled, or soulful, medicine breaks every taboo of Western orthodox medical thinking. The proper and accepted realm of scientific knowledge, as I have discussed above, is the material or physical that we can subject to our detached observation. Dr. George Engel observed how this dogma influences the ways physicians and medical students interact with patients. "Human experience and relating, including dialogue, are outside the scope of scientific knowing and cannot qualify as scientific means of inquiry." Doctors are taught both subtly and directly to see the patient less as a full human being and more as an amalgamation of physical symptoms, a mechanical body constituted by a series of mechanistic processes prone, like a car or a refrigerator, to breaking down.

This vision of the body as a machine, like an automobile prone to breaking down, has profoundly affected the way doctors perceive and care for their patients. Viewing the body as a machine contributes to the dehumanization of the patient–physician relationship and the entire healing process constructed upon that relationship. Not only do doctors tend to treat their patients as mindless, soulless machines, but as physicians become further trained in narrow specialties that compartmentalize the human body, they become accustomed to passing the "patient/machine" down an assembly line of other specialists trained to adjust the smallest of bodily/mechanical functions in remarkable and splendid isolation. Imagining the mechanical body moves us away from our knowledge of the patient as an integrated person and predisposes us too readily to think in terms of "parts" that can be repaired, replaced, or removed.

In the economy of the patient–physician relationship, metaphors of the mechanistic body serve a number of necessities. Obviously, viewing the patient as a machine saves a certain amount of time and energy, which in severe situations, in the emergency room for example, is imperative. In other instances, particularly in the physician's office, there may be so many patients in the waiting room that the doctor has only a few minutes with a patient and therefore must get right down to the specific problem. From the perspective of patients, quick visits may also be appealing in terms of both time and cost of the exam, although findings seem to show that physicians who spend less time with their patients may order more tests to provide further information, and these are always expensive. Not only are these tests costly, the former editor of the *Journal of the American Medical Association* estimates that over half of the *40 million* medical tests ordered *daily* contribute nothing significant to the patient's diagnosis or treatment.

The economics of modern medicine have encouraged physicians to become very poor listeners. Younger physicians and the super specialists seem to be the worst listeners of all doctors. Researchers observed the patient–physician interactions of several doctors and found that, on average, when male physicians ask patients a question they interrupt the patient within eighteen seconds of the reply. The same study showed that fewer than one in fifty patients ever gets to finish a sentence. Female doctors were found to have only slightly better listening skills, waiting an average of thirty-two seconds before interrupting their patients. The former Surgeon General of the United States, C. Everett Koop, has explained this troubling phenomenon in economic terms. Insurance companies pay doctors for procedures and for tests, not for conversation (or "cognitive services").

While machinelike images of the patient may expedite the processes of diagnosis and treatment, they also contain within their mechanistic logic a paradox, exquisitely addressed by Larry Dossey, M.D., in his book *Meaning and Medicine.* Although well-intentioned and caring professionals, physicians who think of their patients as machines may minimize rather than maximize the patient's ability to become well. "Machine models seem always to leave out the qualities that make us quintessentially human."* Our feelings, emotions, beliefs, and souls are what make us quintessentially human, precisely those qualities that physicians are trained to avoid. The metaphor of the machine keeps physicians safe within the realm of the physical body and far removed from the murky terrain of the soul. By dehumanizing the body, we distance ourselves from the essence of what constitutes our humanity—*the soul*—and instead deal solely at the physical level of observable symptoms.

Mechanized Medicine

Do the metaphors, or the pictures in your doctor's mind, matter? Are the metaphors in your physician's head insignificant? Don't you just really care about the treatment that your doctor is capable of providing? This is *precisely* why you should be interested in metaphors of medicine and the way that *your* doctor thinks.

The paths of treatment that physicians follow are charted by their notions of the human body. If your doctor likens your body to a machine, she or he is likely to respond to your illness with mechanical treatments and expect your body to respond accordingly—the way we expect the whole car to run better when we've replaced a corroded battery or replenished its assorted fluids. On the other hand, if your doctor addresses you not merely as a mechanical body of movable parts but as an integrated, whole being, his or her medical response will be more integrated, less invasive and mechanical, and more balanced—more *soulful.*

Orthodox medicine deals most comfortably in mechanical therapies and has historically rejected therapies that appear to work but cannot be explained within the traditional mechanistic map of the body and disease. The UCLA medical team caring for the late Norman Cousins was not prepared for Cousins's self-directed recovery, one of the most celebrated and inspiring triumphs over illness in our time. Checking himself out of the hospital, Cousins replaced his medications with regular doses of vitamin C, the Marx Brothers, and Woody Allen. When his condition improved, the doctors downplayed the powerful role played by Cousins's will to live and his capacity for wholehearted laughter in the face of trauma. Perhaps, they reasoned, he had been misdiagnosed. Perhaps the medication had already delivered its effect before it was stopped. Or maybe the uncommon disease

---

*Larry Dossey, *Meaning and Medicine* (New York: Bantam Books, 1991), 127.

had a naturally limited life span. A favored explanation in baffling cases such as Cousins's is to attribute the healing to a "dummy effect," otherwise known as the placebo effect, the medical term denoting the power of a patient's faith in his or her medical treatment.

Dummy Effects or Superintelligence?

To explain away this recovery as the result of a dummy effect is to insult and diminish the superintelligence of the body's inner Healing Force. The role played by feelings and emotions has been adamantly dismissed by physicians for some time but can no longer be underestimated. Thoughts, feelings, and emotions have been shown to have a powerful influence on many common illnesses, including

- allergies
- asthma
- arthritis
- angina
- hypertension
- acne, psoriasis, hives, and eczema
- irritable bowel, ulcers, colitis, and esophagitis
- migraine and tension headache
- backache and lumbar-sacral sprain
- cancer

The overriding practice in modern medicine is to repudiate cures that are beyond mechanistic explanations. Dr. Larry Dossey notes that "the dominant message, incessantly preached from the editorial pages of medical journals and the podiums of medical schools, is that the 'inherent biology of the disease' is overwhelmingly important and that feelings, emotions, and attitudes are simply along for the ride.'"* In the medical field this amounts to disregarding and discarding hope, faith, and the soul's will to live. Doctors tend to treat such attributes as inconsequential to the healing process. If your body really were just like a car, as the metaphor goes, your feelings and emotions would certainly be riding in the backseat. This approach limits the healing process by diminishing the powerful inner resources that can be summoned to nourish this process along.

---

*Dossey, *Meaning and Medicine*, 133.

At the same time that placebo effects are dismissed as scientifically unexplainable, and therefore seemingly unimportant, the whole foundation of medical research rests upon the mystery of the placebo! This mystery underlies the U.S. Food and Drug Administration's rigorous testing methods that all new drugs must go through. Standard protocol is to randomly divide patients into two groups, one given the drug under consideration, the other, a placebo, or dummy medication, usually nothing more than a sugar pill that looks identical to the drug. Neither the patient nor the physician knows which group receives the real medication, since this information might cloud the outcome of the study. Such a process, it is assumed, allows "objective" evidence that any effects were due to the drug under study. Improvements appearing in patients taking the sugar pill are attributed to their belief in the effectiveness of the treatment they are receiving. Although we cannot explain this phenomenon in our current medical discourse, it is becoming increasingly difficult to dismiss it or belittle its significant and powerful role in the process of healing.

No physician can administer or prescribe the faith and belief underlying such effects. But your doctor can encourage you to draw upon your personal hope and belief and direct it toward the goal of improving your health—making you an active participant in your ongoing healing process. Physicians will be able to do this only if they can learn to feel more comfortable with what they cannot explain. It also requires that patients loosen their expectations that their physician knows everything. Years of medical training and clinical experience instill a deep intelligence in physicians, and a patient's faith in his or her physician's intelligence and skill is an important element in the course of treating illness. But both physicians and patients ought to keep firmly in mind that there is a greater intelligence, a *superintelligence*, within every human, and that this greater intelligence governs the entire process of healing.

ROOM FOR THE SOUL

These days, when matters of the soul do emerge within the walls of Western hospitals, it is typically in the context of a dying patient. It is as if, at these moments, the patient moves to the final stage along the health-care assembly line: the hospital chaplain. When physicians of a terminally ill patient determine there is nothing more that medical science can do to slow the process of necrosis, or the breaking down and dying of the body/

machine, the traditional practice in Western hospitals has been to call a priest, minister, or rabbi to the patient's bedside. The religious professional picks up where the doctor's training ends. We summon these spiritual sources of healing only after we give up on our medical methods. In many hospitals around the country, even this practice occurs less and less. The patient's soul is literally slipping beneath the hospital sheets. *Soulful medicine takes seriously both the pain in the body and the turmoil in the soul and recognizes the interplay between them.*

Searching for the Soul in Science

In historical perspective, the wedge that the medical establishment has driven between the body and the soul is a relatively new turn. In fact, the cultivation of the entire self—body and soul—is actually an ancient motif with its origins in early Greek culture. The ancient physician Seneca embraced the Epicurean principles of the soul in his own writings: "When a man takes care of his body and of his soul, weaving the texture of his good from both, his condition is perfect, and he has found the consummation of his prayers, if there is no commotion in his soul or pain in his body." Seneca spoke of the soul as the "best part" of a person, the source of health and happiness, and therefore worthy of great attention and care.

Drawing on that ancient wisdom, in our own time Thomas Moore has written that "the great malady of the twentieth century, implicated in all of our troubles and affecting us individually and socially, is 'loss of soul.' "* I believe that the most significant contribution I can make as a physician in the 1990s is to tend to this great malady. This book is written out of that conviction. I have learned during my years of practice that the most direct and successful way for me to help effect healthful changes in my patients is to speak to their best part, to address all illness at the level of the soul as well as in its physical manifestations.

Similarly, this book speaks to the best part of you. It addresses not only the pain in your body but provides specific techniques for settling the commotion in your soul. *Soulful Medicine relies on the best that science has to offer while recognizing that the pursuit of health, in its essence, is a spiritual endeavor.*

It is unfortunate that part of every medical student's required training does not include a seminar on the teachings of our ancient and

---

*Moore, *Care of the Soul,* xi.

Renaissance predecessors. From these teachers, new generations of physicians would relearn the deeper meaning of what it means to *practice* medicine. The *wisest practice* of medicine entails the skill of seeing the patient as more than a complex interaction of symptoms and physiological systems, instead seeing the patient as a human being with a soul.

The great sixteenth-century physician Paracelsus recognized the unity between the science of the body and the science of the soul. He called this unity *nature*. Physicians, he said, are only the "servants of nature, not her master." Therefore, he reasoned, "it behooves medicine to follow the will of nature." Thomas Moore reminds us in his book that Paracelsus' Renaissance colleagues believed that the source of every individual emanates from a star in the sky, a notion apparently embraced by the contemporary physicist Paul Davies, who referred to human beings as "animated stardust."

Patients are more than office visits, medical charts, and hospital stops; they are human beings who share an essential origin, humans who begin life from a brilliant source of energy to which they ultimately return. The good physician, according to Paracelsus, views all illnesses in the "macrocosm outside man" and sees the patient in his or her "whole nature." Tending to a patient's illness, from this perspective, is not possible "without profound knowledge of the outer man, *who is nothing other than heaven and earth.*"

Why Is Soul *a Four-Letter Word?*

PBS journalist Bill Moyers recently went on an inquisitive journey into the cutting-edge world of "psychoneuroimmunology," the body of scientific research exploring the possible neurochemical, psychological, and immunological pathways that connect the mind and body. Among the people he interviewed was Candace Pert, a leading neuroscientist whose research has unraveled some of the mysterious chemical pathways that traverse the body and mind. Perhaps no other scientist has come so close to understanding that mind and body are inseparable. Still, Pert's scientific training has instilled within her a clear hesitation, apparent as she tries to describe the real magic that underlies her discovery. "Remember, I'm a scientist, and in the Western tradition I don't use the word 'spirit.' " The language of Western science limits her ability to explain what seems to be happening in the body. " 'Soul' is a four-letter word in our tradition. The deal was struck with Descartes. We don't invoke that stuff.'"*

---

*Bill Moyers, *Healing and the Mind* (New York: Doubleday, 1993), 182.

And yet it is becoming more and more apparent, through the brilliant research of Pert and her colleagues among others, that our knowledge about the body and healing will be enormously limited until we come to grips with the role played by the word we dare not utter: *soul.*

Just because our medical schools and the excellent physicians that emerge from them have neglected the influence of the soul for centuries does not mean that the influence does not exist and is not powerful. Something that cannot be seen or named can still exist. Indeed, people generally have difficulty seeing that which is always present before their very eyes. If, after all, the soul can be seen, perhaps our vision is clouded or we are looking in the wrong places, expecting to find the wrong things. Would we recognize the soul even if it presented itself to us?

In fact, the soul is always revealing itself, sometimes quietly and inwardly, and at other times more dramatically and visibly. But our insistence on understanding all things rationally, our tendency to overanalyze feelings and emotions that do not answer to the rules of reason or logic, blinds us to the soul's *omnipresence.* Most of us lack the ability to listen and feel the soul's presence within our constantly moving bodies and the cobwebs of thought that clutter our minds like old relics in an overflowing attic.

This, after all, is the great ailment of the twentieth century. It is to this ailment that all of us—physicians and patients—need to tend.

Mending the Divide

It appears as though the deal struck with Descartes is off. Mounting evidence shows a multiplicity of ways in which a patient's mental attitudes and beliefs, as well as spiritual outlook, shape her or his health. It is becoming increasingly difficult for physicians to dismiss the presence of a sophisticated healing mechanism in every human being, yet we lack an understanding of how to describe or even conceptualize this awesome force.

Medical researchers, many of them interviewed in Moyers's book *Healing and the Mind,* have taken phenomenal strides toward charting the patterns that interweave the fabric of the body/mind. The factual evidence showing that the mind and body are in constant communication is vast. Deepak Chopra, physician and author of several books, most recently *Ageless Body, Timeless Mind,* and his esteemed colleagues are claiming confidently that *the mind exists in every cell of the body.* And Bill Moyers, who embarked on his research journey with the restraint characteristic of a scientist—journalism is the only profession that clings more strongly to an ethic of objectivity than science—seems to have lost any doubt he had about the sway our emotions hold over the body. Moyers now incorporates into his own daily life the spiritual and mental practices developed by the health professionals he interviewed. In an article appearing after the publication of his book, Moyers remarked that caring for ourselves "is a philosophical quest, not just a scientific quest."

Certainly, scientists differ according to what they mean when they say the mind exists in all cells of the body—some locate this link in a chemical; others, like Chopra, are willing to speak more abstractly about unity at the level of "energy," a concept this book returns to frequently. While some physicians are acknowledging a connection between the mind and body, others are beginning to suggest that no distinction exists between the body and the mind at all, that they are one and the same.

Advances in what is being called "mind/body medicine" demonstrate that scientists are rethinking that fundamental myth of Western science—the myth of the "divided self," the notion that somehow our body and mind are not the same. We are learning more and more about the integration of body and mind that confronts the limits of our biological, materialistic medicine.

Even our medical language is inadequate to describe these innovations. The name *mind/body* to some extent actually reinforces the divisive thinking set into motion centuries ago by Descartes. Language, in a sense, is limited by and in turn limits the ways we see things. We tend to see the world in terms of binary frameworks, divisions between, for instance, black or white, mind or body, good or bad, and so on. Dividing the human being along the axes of mind and body may make human existence more understandable, but it also obscures its complexity. In reality, the soul encompasses both body and mind and makes them one.

Joan Borysenko, a leader in psychoneuroimmunology research, prefers to speak in terms of the "bodymind," a reference picked up by others, including Chopra. Removing the slash helps heal the division that our language tends to fortify. Robert Ader, a psychologist who has done groundbreaking research in immunology, describes exactly the limitations of our language to help explain the idea that mind and body are inseparable. "We have a one-dimensional language for a three-dimensional concept."* The wisdom of the body does not differentiate between physical and

---

*Moyers, *Healing and the Mind,* 245.

emotional dimensions; why should physicians? Borysenko's rendition is both creative and crucial, for it recognizes this wisdom that joins together the body and the mind.

Paradigm Shift

It is impossible to underestimate the magnitude of importance behind this shift in scientific vision. Fifteen years ago, very few physicians were willing to entertain the thought of a significant relationship between body and mind. Those of us who began to think seriously about the influence of the mind over the body's state were not, in turn, taken seriously by our professional community. But physicians have to take seriously the fact that their patients are turning in large numbers to the so-called alternative healing practices. It is a cause for concern because we must encourage responsible alternatives.

And it is cause for great hope. Physicians who not long ago were ostracized for speaking about the relationship between body and mind are now seeing the seeds of research they planted cultivated on a grander scale by a new generation of scientists, with the slow but increasing approval of the medical establishment. Physicians and medical researchers at renowned institutions, including Harvard, Berkeley, Johns Hopkins, and the Salk Institute, are reconstructing a medicine that can integrate new findings about the workings of the mind to expand our medical knowledge as well as our ability to help our patients heal.

I hope this book will contribute to this grand effort. For even as we extend our medical vision to make room for the mind's influence over the physical body, our ability as physicians to help our patients will be limited until we recognize the expression of the soul behind each physical symptom we attempt to treat.

More and more physicians who are speaking of a mind/body connection are now being ushered into the mainstream. Could it be that in another decade's time *soul* will no longer be a four-letter word? Will physicians who tend to the commotion in a patient's soul as well as cure their physical symptoms of illness soon be respected by their colleagues rather than dismissed, as they too often are? The breakthroughs in body-mind medicine give both patients and their doctors hope that all of this will be true. Scientists seem to be rethinking their ideas about the validity of the soul as a subject of scientific inquiry.

It is only a matter of time before physicians become aware that the final stitch in the suturing of the body/mind split rests with the soul. Western medicine is still governed by the primacy of biology, to be sure. Rather than making a choice between two emphases—body *or* mind—the purpose of this book is to reacquaint you with the essence that is the unity underlying and integrating both. When we reframe our perspective of the biological human being from the standpoint of the soul, we are able to overcome the divisive thinking that has encouraged the artificial division between mind and body for centuries. *The soul encompasses both and makes them singular.* In fact, from the standpoint of the soul such distinctions are meaningless. This is the view of Soulful Medicine. When we recognize this we will finally dismantle the dualistic and mechanistic frameworks in which we view, diagnose, and treat human disease. And we will be a long way on our journey toward wellness.

The Ultimate Cure

By denying the need for healing at the level of the soul, we automatically limit our capacity to get well. The ancient physicians knew, and Thomas Moore has recently reminded us, that "the ultimate cure comes from love and not from logic."[*] The soul expresses itself through love and is the force that renders body and mind inseparable. This underlying, unifying force is gradually gaining recognition by doctors and patients. When pressed by Moyers to provide a precise definition of mind/body medicine, Dr. Dean Ornish responded in a way that recognizes this unifying force: "In a way, mind/body medicine is a kind of misnomer because this kind of healing goes beyond mind and body to some of the psychosocial and even spiritual dimensions."[**] Ornish is among the pioneering physicians of our time who fuses the innovations of modern medicine with the wisdom of the ancient physicians to find a role for the imagination—the language of the soul—in healing.

Many scientists, doctors included, are beginning to speak about a fundamental shift in our ways of knowing and thinking about the world. They call this a "paradigm shift." Today's shift seems to be away from the dualistic mindset inherited from the Enlightenment and toward a more unified theory of science and human existence. Central to this shift are concepts of the soul, nature, and God.

---

[*]Moore, *Care of the Soul,* 14.

[**]Moyers, *Healing and the Mind,* 104.

17

THE WALKING
WOUNDED

My own medical vision began to shift dramatically fifteen years ago. At that time, I was the founder and president of one of the most reputable and busy pediatrics practices in California. By all standard measures, I had achieved success as a physician: my practice was booming, I saw patient after patient, eight hours a day six days a week, and my skills as a diagnostician were widely acclaimed by my professional colleagues.

So why did I feel so incomplete?

During this period I began sensing a disconcerting pattern emerging in my practice. It seemed to me that of all the hundreds of patients I saw each week, those who returned most frequently—ten to twenty times a year—were not the children my medical knowledge lead me to expect would need frequent medical attention. These were not children with leukemia, Down's syndrome, juvenile rheumatoid arthritis, and other inherited immune deficiencies or genetic syndromes.

My appointment book indicated, to my genuine amazement, that the children I was seeing for repeated visits were those with troubling but nonspecific illnesses, including upper respiratory problems such as allergies, wheezing, coughing, congestion; gastrointestinal problems including constipation, diarrhea, colitis, proctitis, and weight problems; skin problems such as rashes, eczema, and psoriasis; and repeat infections of otitis, tonsillitis, bronchitis, sinusitis, and pyelonephritis.

Together, these wheezing, coughing, sniffling, itchy children constituted just 20 percent of my practice. Analysis of the appointment charts and financial ledgers revealed a truly shocking pattern: *20 percent of my patients were sick 80 percent of the time.* In other words, 20 percent of my patients were utilizing 80 percent of my professional hours and generating 80 percent of my income!

However much I wanted to resist these findings, the implications were inescapable. My entire view of illness and disease, my knowledge of how to practice medicine, my understanding of the patient-physician relationship—all of this had to change, even though I was thinking and doing *exactly* what I learned in medical school and my clinical training.

I began to spend my time with that troubling 20 percent differently. I wanted to learn more about them and the sources of their illnesses. I kept my prescription pad tucked deep in my doctor's coat, and before I even reached for my stethoscope, I began talking to the children and their parents. I learned to listen to, not just *hear*, their stories, not just the facts of their medical histories, but their thoughts, beliefs, and feelings about illness.

Listening to my patients and their parents talk about why they thought illness was returning again and again, it became apparent to me that somewhere, somehow, the seed of one debilitating thought had been planted and was now growing out of control like a tenacious weed. That thought is this: illness is natural, inevitable, something to expect.

This is not to suggest that the parents of these perpetually ill children did not want their children to be healthy. These parents truly thought that an important part of being a good parent was protecting their children from illness. Of course, they were right. But the frequent presence of illness in their children's lives suggested to me that this outlook, when carried to the extreme point where parents actively feared and geared up for the next illness, was actually contributing to the frequency of illness their children experienced.

A LESSON ANY GRANDMOTHER WOULD UNDERSTAND

What I was seeing was really a version of the same phenomenon I experienced when I was a child in the Bronx. Each time I went outside to play, without fail my grandmother stood by the door admonishing me lovingly as she handed me my hat and gloves: "Eddie boy, you're going to catch a cold." She knew everything; why should she be wrong about this? My grandmother expected me to get sick, and she was so convincing that over time I internalized this worry and expectation. To this day I remind myself each time I step out into even the slightest chilly morning that if I don't bundle up I will catch a cold. Do we catch colds because we expose ourselves to harsh weather, or is it our expectation that when we do so we will catch a cold that actually brings on the first sniffle?

I came to describe people in this state of worry and expectation as the "Worried Well and the Walking Wounded." When their children had no symptoms of illness or discomfort, these parents worried and geared up for the next onset of illness.

One afternoon, a nurse saw me brooding over my patients' charts. I had given them the best medical and diagnostic treatment possible, and yet they were perpetually ill for apparently no reason except that they lived in environments where illness was expected. How could I go on treating their minor sniffles and rashes without addressing this underlying problem? Eight years of medical training had not prepared me for the despair I felt over this. The nurse asked a question that immediately shifted my perspective on what I was convinced were depressing statistics. "What about the other 80 percent of your patients? Why aren't they getting sick?"

If a destructive attitude about illness was the common thread connecting the 20 percent of my patients whom I called the Worried Well and the Walking Wounded, was a different attitude shared among the families whose babies and children were well? I began to explore the lessons to be learned from the 80 percent of my patients who took up so little of my office visits, coming to see me only for checkups and school physicals. Surely enough, what distinguished them from the "Worried Well" was that the weedlike thought that illness is inevitable simply had not been planted in their minds, or if it existed there once, it had since been firmly uprooted.

The parents of these children did not expect them to be sick, but neither did they adopt a hopeless attitude on the infrequent occasions when they were sick. It was more than the absence of a negative health outlook that characterized these families; the parents of these children simply had no time for illness given their active lifestyles. This was true across distinctions based on race and class. These families did not make room for illness in their lives. As a group, however, these families tended to incorporate a host of "well choices" that influenced their healthy lives: most of these parents did not smoke and only a very few had problems with alcohol or drugs; most parents and their children were within the normal range of weight; and many of these families shared core spiritual beliefs or values that connected them to an extended family or local community, whether through a church, synagogue, or other kind of support network.

Your "Soul" Purpose Is to Be Well

These parents were teaching their children and their physician—myself—an important life lesson: health is determined less by genes and medicine than it is shaped by an attitude characterized by three crucial factors: SELF-VALUE, PERSONAL RESPONSIBILITY, and REVERENCE FOR LIFE.

The "Worried Well" confronted me with a profound professional and personal choice concerning their treatment. The orthodox approach, from the physician's perspective, was to continue treating the symptoms of illness by administering the appropriate medications and injections with an occasional dietary recommendation as a passing thought. But looking at their medical charts made it absolutely clear that the standard approach would provide temporary treatment at best. In one or two months' time, the same patients were likely to return with many of the same symptoms, as they had before.

My second option was to apply the lessons learned from those patients and their children so seldom seen in my office. Such a treatment would need to address the deeper aches and ailments underlying their array of physical symptoms. Barring any major physical problem, immune deficiency, or inherited genetic syndrome, which I ruled out immediately, why else would these physical symptoms keep recurring if there were not some deeper ailment—a soul sickness—not being addressed by the pre-scribed medication?

Although I had a superior understanding of *how* the illnesses were occurring and what medications would halt further progression of the specific illness; what my reliance on scientific reason was blinding me to was an understanding of *why* the illnesses were occurring in the first place and with such startling frequency. My professional preoccupation with the mechanics of illness was stifling my ability to interpret the *meaning* of illness.

When I began looking at illness in the broader context of the patient's attitudes, behaviors, and family relationships, it became apparent that any lasting treatment would need to attend to these factors as well as the physical symptoms. Such treatment involved the entire family and might include asking parents to do the following:

- stop smoking
- stop using spanking as a form of punishment
- openly praise and love their children more
- turn off the TV and encourage children to play outdoors
- eat less red meat and junk food
- practice stress-reversal or relaxation techniques

In short, I needed to reenlist my patients and their families for the long haul, to recharge their self-value, motivate their personal responsibility, and replace a "just getting by" attitude with the excitement of staying well or getting well, a profound and enthusiastic reverence for life. Before issuing any more prescriptions, before administering any more penicillin shots, I needed to create a bridge to deliver my patients from the illness-is-to-be-expected outlook to the experience of a timeless truth: against all physical odds, *your "soul" purpose is to be well.*

WELLNESS WITHIN

Initially, I did not realize the powerful strength and tenacity of the self-destructive thought that illness is to be expected. My first approach to reeducate my patients and their parents reflected my own deeply entrenched reliance on mechanistic models of the body and health. Imagine how absurd the following directions for learning to walk would seem: first, lift your right foot, bending slightly at the knee, and use your hip muscle to propel you forward as you lower the right foot while simultaneously beginning this motion again with the left foot. Of course this makes no sense. Even if we could explain walking in a reasonably simple and reductive manner to an infant, he or she would not have the language skills to comprehend our instructions. An infant learns to walk through experience: the experience of observing others around her in motion; the (generally) successive experiences of crawling, standing, and eventually taking a few steps toward mother or father before tumbling to her knees.

Learning that *your "soul" purpose is to be well* works the same way, through experience. I learned quickly that the Walking Wounded could not be mechanically taught this lesson, as if the information would enter one end of the machine and put the "gears" in motion. There I was, in my lab coat with diagrams in hand, trying to apply rational scientific discourse to a matter totally inaccessible to our stubborn intellects. Showing a diagram of overlapping circles consisting of "body," "mind," and "soul" with arrows charting various flows of interactions among the components was about as effective as presenting an infant with a pattern of the foot positions required to move from one end of the room to the other.

This is not to suggest that these parents lacked the intelligence to understand my diagrams; quite the opposite. It is to reveal instead my own limited framework for thinking about and describing the process of achieving balanced, soulful health. My charts and diagrams were clumsy at best, confusing at worst.

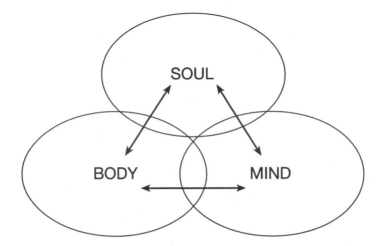

The wellness that comes from within—soul wellness—cannot very well be charted in a linear or logical fashion. This inner wellness must be experienced. Difficult to imagine or explain, once you have felt its presence, you will never think of your health in the same way again. Nothing can compare with what you will experience through practicing the very same meditation I taught to the Walking Wounded—many of them children as young as four years old. You will experience firsthand the soul's presence as it expands throughout your body. By doing nothing more than quieting your mind, stilling your body, and calming your breath, you will be able to coax the soul's Healing Force to announce its presence and render its healing influence. Please take a moment to contemplate this simple meditation that begins with seven long slow breaths. Be still and practice the meditation dwelling on a different message at this time. Substitute "God loves me . . . God loves me . . . God loves me" for "I am loved."

Meditation Technique
Practicing the Presence of Peace

- Close your eyes and consciously relax your breathing. Breathe naturally, through your nose, and with each breath draw in a feeling of peace and calm.

- Now, take a long, even relaxed breath and as you exhale relax your forehead and the muscles behind your eyes.

- Take a long, even relaxed breath and as you exhale release the tension around your mouth, jaw and neck.

- Take a long, even relaxed breath and as you exhale relax your shoulders, arms, hands and fingers.

- Take a long, even relaxed breath and as you exhale let go of the tension in your chest and abdomen.

- Take a long, even relaxed breath and as you exhale relax the muscles throughout your back and buttocks.

- Take a long, even relaxed breath and as you exhale release the tension in your thighs, calves, feet and toes.

- Take a long, even relaxed breath and as you exhale picture a radiant golden healing light filling your entire body from your toes to the very tip of your head.

- Continue to breathe slowly and deeply and inwardly affirm over and over to yourself: I am loved . . . I am loved . . . I am loved . . . I am loved . . . I am loved.

- Continue repeating this for as long as you wish. Before finishing, sit quietly for a moment, eyes closed, feeling the presence of peace permeating every cell of your body.

UNDERSTANDING ILLNESS

When I first opened the Wellness Medical Institute in Mt. Carmel, Illinois, I placed a notice in the newspapers announcing a new phase of health care that Hippocrates would approve. The announcement listed my medical credentials, special training, and the hours and location of my new family and pediatric practice. I also included the following statement: "As a wellness-minded physician, I am committed to spending as much time discerning why your disease occurs as I spend on diagnosis and medical treatment of the physical symptoms of that disease." I offered consultative services for a wide variety of conditions including anxiety, depression, stress, headache, backache, hypertension, chronic fatigue, insomnia, and addictions.

My first patient was Anne Myers, a fifty-nine-year-old woman whose first words to me were: "Doctor, I have everything in your announcement." Indeed, Anne's medical history revealed that since she had a hysterectomy ten years earlier for dysfunctional uterine bleeding, she suffered from literally every symptom listed in my newspaper notice and then some. Anne had seen at least eight doctors in the surrounding area and was currently being treated for chronic fatigue syndrome by a local physician.

Reading Anne's medical charts produced during the nine years since her hysterectomy, I could not help but think they sounded like a virtual "hunt" for a physical cause of her symptoms. Anne's problems were first diagnosed as mitral valve prolapse, then as subclinical panic disorder, then as "yeast syndrome," and after that it was hypoglycemia, environmental and food allergy, depression, and finally, chronic fatigue syndrome. She had been taking combinations of Ativan, Prozac, Zoloft, and Valium for the last nine years. Despite the potency of each of these drugs, Anne had no relief of her symptoms.

We talked for a while about her personal history, since nothing in her official medical history was particularly revealing about her condition. Anne had married a coal miner she met while attending a junior college in the area thirty years ago. The last eight years had been marked by increasing anger and marital strife. She had two daughters and three grandchildren who lived nearby. Family get-togethers were essentially limited to holidays because "no one really gets along well together." Anne had no brothers or sisters and remembers her mother constantly lamenting the fact that she had never had a son. Her mother died of breast cancer at age fifty-one, her father of lung cancer at age sixty-five. Both parents were heavy smokers. So were her daughters and her husband.

Like her family members, Anne smoked "about two packs a day." She also drank more than a full pot of coffee daily and avoided all forms of exercise. She watched television about five hours a day, mostly news, soap operas, and talk shows, and in between she took naps because of exhaustion. Anne's diet consisted mainly of lots of red meat: bacon for breakfast, ham or bologna for lunch, and hamburger or pork chops for dinner.

Anne's physical examination revealed an expressionless face compatible with clinical depression, and she appeared to be exhausted but without any alarming or specific abnormalities. Her blood pressure was slightly elevated (140 over 90), but examination of her heart and peripheral circulation showed them to be normal. Although she coughed frequently, examination of her throat, sinuses, and lungs was unrevealing. A slight fine tremor in both hands was present; however, her neurological examination, including the cranial nerves, was entirely normal, and her thyroid gland was not remarkable. Examination of her abdomen was normal, and a pelvic exam revealed an absent uterus and cervix.

A number of diagnoses had previously been made by a host of physicians, who prescribed a number of potent drugs for Anne. Most of these medications probably had the unintended side effect of just compounding Anne's weariness, but none of the medications even brushed the surface of the source of her exhaustion.

After my examination and an hour-long consultation it appeared evident to me that the patient's chronic fatigue was a physical symptom of a deeper illness that would require an entirely different medical approach. The key to Anne's wellness would clearly have to be a personal commitment on her part to make several significant lifestyle changes.

No medicine was going to provide a remedy for all that ailed her, and there was essentially nothing more I could add to Anne's previous diagnoses, and I told her so. But I emphasized that there was ample reason to believe that with proper care and a well-thought-out strategy she could restore the quality and vitality so sorely lacking in her life. Anne enthusiastically proclaimed her total willingness, saying: "Doctor Taub, I want you to know that I will do anything to feel better."

Clearly the smoking, caffeine, high-fat diet, and aversion to exercise were necessary targets for lifestyle change. I asked her, as I have asked you in this book, to embark on a journey toward wellness. I described this journey to Anne as an inward passage, self-motivated and self-directed. No packing, no passport, no travel required. What the journey does require, I explained, is a personal commitment to restoring vibrant energy in one's life. Anne seemed anxious to make this commitment.

I left the examination room for a moment to confer with my nurse, who would be filling Anne in on the details of her treatment. "Be very patient and understanding with Anne. Try to deal with any resistance that she offers by suggesting a compromise. She is a long-suffering person." My nurse entered the room and began to "administer" the Wellness Rx, a discussion and question-and-answer process that usually takes about thirty minutes. After just ten minutes, my nurse stopped me in the hallway between examining rooms to explain that Anne was willing to make a verbal promise to follow the Wellness Rx, but she would not agree to sign the written promise that would become part of her medical chart.

Puzzled, I followed the nurse back into the examination room, to find Anne standing in the middle of the room, poised to leave with her hands firmly placed on her hips.

"You have no right to insinuate that I can't keep my word!" Anne's voice was shaky.

"But Anne, this is only a promise you make to yourself. Signing the patient agreement only seals the promise," I explained, without much effect.

"I *will* promise, Doctor, to do everything in this Wellness Rx, but I *won't* sign it. And that's that!"

Reluctantly, for the first time ever encountering this type of opposition from a patient, I conceded to a verbal promise from Anne. I didn't feel comfortable about the compromise at all.

Anne returned one week later. When I asked her how she was feeling, she seemed resigned.

"You were right," she said. "I couldn't stick with it." "It" referred to just about everything in the prescription. "I need beef to feel right. Meditating annoys me. And just thinking of the brisk walk you asked me to take made my blood pressure elevate. Also, I can't do without my coffee."

We stared at each other for a long moment, neither one of us knowing quite what to say. Anne filled the silence with more than a hint of discouragement.

"So it's not worth it to me."

"What *would* your wellness be worth?" I asked.

Anne's mind seemed elsewhere, busy. Finally, she pushed the patient agreement aside and stood up, saying, "I figured out that it's not necessary for me to do the things you asked. It finally dawned on me that I must have allergies to the environment and I just have to learn to live with it." Anne thanked me for my interest and walked out of my office smiling.

It's discouraging when your efforts to reach someone and help them are in vain. When I got over the disappointment of losing Anne's interest I began to understand some important reasons for her suffering. Why hadn't I noticed the link between Anne's hysterectomy and the physical symptoms plaguing her since her surgery, earlier?

The first signs of exhaustion had appeared within six months of Anne's surgery. While the hysterectomy addressed the bleeding problem, it clearly did not address the underlying energy imbalance causing the problem in the first place. Indeed, surgery may have tilted her energy scales so far off balance that a variety of symptoms, some minor, some serious, were invoked. To recall the musical analogy introduced in a previous chapter, even if you remove a troublesome E string from a violin, its absence still disrupts the sound energy generated from the instrument. Of course, it's easier to replace an E string than an internal organ. Although the uterus cannot be replaced, the energy imbalance caused by its removal can be addressed on another level.

The loss of any vital organ traumatizes the rest of the body, and all parts of the body may respond to this absence. Unfortunately, the medical establishment tends to regard the uterus as "disposable." Hysterectomy (literally, "removal of the womb") is the second most frequently performed major surgery in the United States, despite the troubling fact that the majority of doctors would only agree with the necessity of the operation just *10 percent* of the time. The widespread attitude exists among doctors that the uterus exists only to house the fetus during pregnancy. From a strictly mechanical standpoint, this is true. But such a notion is incoherent or inconceivable from the perspective that your body is energy. The uterus, like all other organs, plays a role in maintaining the balanced flow of energy to all aspects of the body. Depression after any major surgery is not unusual; in the case of hysterectomy, prolonged depression or fatigue is common, depending on the emotional support a woman receives from friends, family, and her physician.

Not made aware of alternative therapies to surgery, Anne established a gloomy and potentially devastating outlook on illness. Consciously or unconsciously, from any number of sources including doctors, parents, friends, and the media, Anne was programmed to believe that *illness is cured by removing the affected tissue or organ*. But if this were true, why would Anne still have so many illnesses after her "problem" uterus was removed?

Anne appears to be on the threshold of perennial fatigue because neither she nor her staff of physicians could locate and excise the source of her weariness. With no such outlet, Anne adopted an immobilizing attitude: "I'll just have to learn to live with the illness." She identified so strongly with her illnesses that the idea of actually living without them threatened her very sense of self. She was prepared to defend her illnesses (or dismiss them as incurable food allergies) and the life she had developed around them. For a person who feels ceaselessly tired, it is not hard to see why this "learn to live with it" outlook is more easily adopted than the Nike™-inspired "just-do-it" mentality embedded in our popular culture these days.

Like the body, the soul requires nourishment and care, without which it too will become weary and depressed. The soul is a bit like a stubborn pet who becomes a nuisance for want of its caretaker's attention. Chewing up a shoe or emptying the kitchen trash while its master is away is really a sign that says, "I'm hungry for love and play. You're neglecting me. Pay attention to me!" Exhaustion, high blood pressure, teariness, and depression are cries from the soul for more attention. If we ignore these soul cries for too long the soul itself becomes undernourished and cannot provide the vitality and joy that are essential to living.

The burdens of our beliefs chain us to our illusions of illness. Anne's symptoms of chronic fatigue are dramatic expressions of the soul's hunger for care. And yet she is convinced that she is too tired to make any personal change that requires effort. Instead of learning to *live* with her symptoms, Anne needs to learn how to *listen* to what her symptoms reveal.

In *Care of the Soul,* Thomas Moore identifies depression, exhaustion, a hunger for joy and happiness as symptoms that speak of a "loss of soul." These symptoms, according to Moore, reveal to us what the soul craves. Instead of thinking of illness as an isolated occurrence that needs to be excised from the body, from the perspective of the soul we can look at all disease and discomfort in the broader personal, emotional, and social context of the person. When we learn to think in this way, we can begin to decode the signs that symptoms of depression and fatigue present and begin the process of transformation that they call for.

Anne was raised to believe that her mission in life was to bear and raise children. Since she had accomplished this with success, she was led to believe that her productive life was over, her contribution made. While hysterectomy brings closure to a woman's *r*eproductive life, it certainly does not mean her *productive* life has ended. Yet for Anne, coming of age in a time and town where a woman's worth was tied to reproduction, life lost its meaning and purpose shortly after surgery. The human body quickly responds to a loss of meaning. Illnesses like Anne's reveal this loss.

A Word About Genes

> *We should be careful about the meaning we allow "gene"*
> *and "genetic" to hold for us, for these meanings determine*
> *what we deem to be possible, and can either enhance or*
> *interfere with healing.*
> —*Larry Dossey, M.D.*

Interpreting illness as soul-sickness and energy imbalance does not mean that genetics play no role. However, Soulful Medicine reassesses science's reliance on DNA as the source of all disease and acknowledges the deeper meaning behind illness. Let me illustrate this through the experiences of another patient, a thirty-seven-year-old woman, Rachel Barnes.

Rachel was struggling to overcome a seven-year period in which she had been experiencing blindingly severe migraine headaches. In the past six months, the migraines had become so severe that they carried her into a bout of disabling depression. Under my medical care for nearly a month, Rachel confided in me that she was beginning to give in to hopelessness. Although improved nutrition, meditation, and regular light exercise had improved her outward appearance, inside she still felt lifeless. Beta blockers and antidepressant medication were providing no relief for Rachel's migraines, and the headaches were forcing her into increasing isolation. The darkness of her bedroom was only a small comfort. There was nothing her family could do to make her feel any more at ease.

I was proposing a change in her treatment plan when Rachel interrupted.

"I appreciate your interest and care, Doctor. But I feel I'm wasting your time. Let's face it. You just can't fight genetics."

I assured Rachel that while migraine and depression have a genetic component, the problems she was experiencing could still be overcome. Looking over her medical records, I further remarked that there was no mention of any diseases in her family. Her records indicated that both parents died of natural causes related to aging. There was no apparent history of diabetes, cancer, tuberculosis, or inherited disease. "These are good signs," I told the patient.

"Doctor, you don't understand. My grandmother, mother, and sister have all had breast cancer. I must have it too." Rachel was growing visibly upset.

As we continued to speak openly, it became clear that my patient was experiencing a deepening depression because she thought she would soon lose her breast, if not her life. "You have no lumps or bumps, no masses, nodules, cysts, discoloration, or discharge. Your mammogram is entirely normal." I tried to explain that even if abnormalities were present, there are many treatments that were not available to her grandmother or even her mother. "But why didn't you tell me or any of your other doctors about your family history?"

Rachel shrugged. The very thought of treatment paralyzed her. "But, Rachel, there aren't any lumps now."

Her reply was revealing: "But the genes are there!"

Rachel learned what most of us were taught in our high school biology classes. Genes determine our destiny. Rachel's migraines and depression finally disappeared when she came to recognize how false and potentially life-threatening this reductive view can be. If you were destined to live and die by your genes, in fact every one of us would suffer thousands of diseases for as long as we lived—which would not be so long!

DNA is a powerful determinant in your health. But the power of genes to determine disease is not unlimited, and that power is not beyond the influence of important factors that are within your control.

The primary factors shaping your health are personal responsibility, self-value, and reverence for life. Your DNA, though it contains all of the diseases and weaknesses inherited from your mother, father, grandparents, on up the family tree, remains in balance for most of your life. Although the genetic blueprints, or templates, of almost all of the diseases of all of your ancestors are encoded in your DNA, you are generally without these illnesses most of your life. If genes are your destiny, why don't you develop your great-grandmother's rheumatoid arthritis, your grandfather's prostate cancer, your mother's diabetes, your father's hypertension, and so on?

Blueprints of Disease

The reason you are not a perpetual walking genetic disaster is because your natural inner resources maintain your body's equilibrium and harmony. The current scientific explanation of this phenomenon hinges on a substance called suppressor RNA and its role in the dynamic network of intelligence that is your genetic structure. Suppressor RNA is able to block the transport of encoded template messages by messenger RNA, which is the substance that piggybacks genetic messages to the powerhouses of your cells that manufacture proteins according to these genetic messages. Suppressor RNA blocks the delivery of disease templates and blueprints inherited from your ancestors. Rachel was basically healthy and much too young for the natural processes of aging to be unlocking any templates of disease inherited from her ancestors.

The textbook scientific explanation of DNA ends here, but from the perspective of energy and wellness, this process answers to a higher intelligence: the Healing Force. The codes or blueprints of disease in your DNA are under the sway of your every attitude and behavior. The way you think and feel and the choices of action that you take either enhance or impede the Healing Force's ability to keep disease at bay. Your inner healer is like a gatekeeper, keeping these templates of disease safely stored away. When the flow of the Healing Force is obstructed, when the body's energy is out of balance, the templates of disease pry through the gates that normally keep them at a safe distance.

Research has demonstrated the powerful effect that emotions, beliefs, and attitudes have on genetic processes. Researchers at Ohio State have observed that DNA repair—the built-in capacity of DNA to repair its own mistakes with special enzymes—was significantly poorer in highly depressed patients than in patients with mild depression. DNA repair in healthy adults without depression was superior to both depressed groups. If poor mental outlook weakens the immunological processes controlled by DNA, then mental vitality and soul strength can enhance the productivity of these biochemical healers.

Only when the templates of disease are unleashed is the risk of developing an inherited disease present. Your efforts, then, must be to enhance your body's inner resolve to keep these templates safely stored away. If they have already been unlocked, then you must learn ways to bolster your body's innate healing responses, which are powerful enough to neutralize the destructive force of disease. Rachel's misperception was that if the genetic predisposition for breast cancer were present in her body, so was the actual disease. She felt helpless because she thought her genes had absolute authority over her health destiny. This perspective is thoroughly diffused by Dr. Dossey, who casts a different focus on the issue of genetics. *"People suffering from genetic diseases need not change the genes themselves, only their manifestations."* * Rachel's prolonged suffering of migraine and depression may very well have had the power to unlock the templates of breast cancer she shares with other women in her family. But the power of her Healing Force is greater, and she no longer experiences migraine or depression. When Rachel dismantled the architecture of her attitudes, her belief that genes reign supreme when it comes to disease, she removed a major barrier from the flow of the Healing Force that promises to keep her well.

More important than the genes that you inherit are the beliefs you inherit. Your assumptions and expectations about illness have as much sway over your health as your genetic makeup. If you treat genes as your destiny, they become destiny. It is your interpretation of their power that gives genes power over your health. It is possible to willfully summon your own Healing Force to fight life-destroying genetic patterns. Your belief, as Norman Cousins illustrated, can become your biology. Before learning ways of changing your beliefs about illness, not merely to ward off disease but to live life with reverence and joy, let's first look more closely at disease itself.

---

*Larry Dossey, *Meaning and Medicine*, 154. Italics in original.

Decoding Disease

The idea that disease is a physical manifestation of an imbalance in the body's energy is as old as medicine itself. The genealogy of this idea was recently traced in an article in the *Journal of the American Medical Association*. Nearly three thousand years ago, Empedocles theorized that all matter is composed of dynamically opposed elements, or energy, and that balance and harmony are essential to human survival. Hippocrates elaborated on these ideas a century later, describing health as the harmonious balance of forces. Disease, according to Hippocrates' model, is the equivalent of dissonance, or the breakdown of harmony in the elements of the human system. In the nineteenth century, Claude Bernard coined the phrase *milieu interieur* to refer to this innate harmonious equilibrium. The esteemed twentieth-century physiologist Walter Cannon, responsible for the term *homeostasis*, described an interior harmony that involves emotional as well as physical elements.

So you see that the understanding of disease as energy imbalance has been evolving for nearly three millennia. In each century, the essential idea that health is the presence of harmony and balance of physical, mental, and emotional forces in the body has been refined and filtered through the beliefs of a given culture at a given historical moment. In our own medical culture, governed by the imperatives of a profit-driven insurance industry, corporate ownership of hospitals, high technology, and the mechanical logic of disease repair, this belief has become so diluted as to almost be forgotten. But just because medicine has forgotten about the healing power within us does not mean that it no longer exists.

The task of this book is to remind you about homeostasis, and to provide you with the tools to restore and reinvigorate that harmonious balance which is wellness. When you have felt this inner balance for the briefest of moments, the memory of that feeling will guide you in your journey toward wellness and nurture your resolve to listen to what your body's symptoms have to tell you about your soul.

The Hidden Roots of Disease

The reason why medications and surgical procedures often do little more than temporarily relieve our symptoms of disease is because these techniques fail to dislodge the deeper roots of disease. Every illness, physical or mental, is anchored in our perception. Our assumptions and expectations of disease are the sediment in which disease buries its anchors.

When it comes to our outlook on illness, our minds are like overgrown gardens. Destructive thoughts about illness clutter the gardens of our minds like unruly and tenacious weeds. These thought-weeds crowd out the would-be flowers of thought that inspire good health and inner balance. Even the tallest sunflower cannot stretch toward the sun when it is burdened by so many weeds.

Belief Becomes Biology

If we were to make our way through some of these mental weeds, we would arrive at a series of thoughts, attitudes, and assumptions about illness and disease. These beliefs are like mental blueprints that literally map the paths and routes that illness follows. Identifying the presence of these mental blueprints helps us map not only where and how our illnesses emerged but also our journey back to wellness. Where the seeds of these thoughts came from and how they took root in our minds depend on the specific circumstances of the person and the role played by illness in his or her lifetime. I know that one of my most powerful assumptions was planted in my mind by my grandmother: "If you go out in the cold and your hair gets wet you'll get sick." She probably inherited this thought from her grandmother. Our family is one source of the beliefs we hold about disease.

Attitudes toward illness are also programmed by the advertising campaigns of the multibillion-dollar pharmaceutical industry. One recent commercial features a man suffering from an upset stomache as he struggles to squeeze his legs into a yoga posture in one scene and looks sadly at a plate with a few peas and a string of pasta in the next. A comforting voice-over asks, "Why change your lifestyle when you can take Rolaids®?"

Our minds are programmed to be ill and to depend on medication from a very early age. We are taught that it is easier to medicate an illness than to change the behaviors that may have illicited the illness in the first place. The overt message behind all of these illness-inducing thoughts is that when it comes to being sick, we have no choice. We have been conditioned over generations and generations to believe that illness is inevitable and that the best we can do is medicate our bodies while we ride out the next wave of illness. The barrage of media messages would lead us all to believe we have no choice but to dive in.

Think for a moment about the strands of your own mental blueprints. How did your parents respond when they got sick? When you had a cold, how did your mother or father take care of you? What did you learn about caring for a cold? What did illness mean to you when you

were a child? A day or two off from school? A few more hours in front of
the television set? Chicken soup? The opportunity to stay in your pajamas
all day? A new toy or gift from a sympathetic parent? Or was illness an
unwelcomed guest that kept you off the playground? Was a cold a
nuisance because you couldn't join the rest of the kids in snowball fights
and making snow angels?

The thoughts learned in the past may seem inconsequential to the
journey you are about to embark upon toward wellness. Quite the opposite, however, these memories are the pathways of your mental condition-
ing. Too often they lead directly to the thought: "I must be getting sick."
This self-defeating thought actually sets into motion a whole sequence of
physiological events as the nervous system "gears up" for the approaching
illness. Just the thought "I must be getting sick" triggers the body's
generalized adaptive response to stress, a process first described by Dr.
Hans Selye. One small thought causes the body's natural steroids to rise,
produces a change in blood cell properties, puts the entire central, endo-
crine and immune systems on alert, sending up an internal red flag of
imminent danger. Every thought, no matter how fleeting, unleashes a
messenger molecule in your brain that triggers a physiological response.
The illnesses you endure, each and every one of them, to a much larger
extent than was once imagined, is the product of how you perceive health.
Anxious ideas about the inevitability of a cold in winter are invitations to
illness. So is the expectation that because your mother and your sister had
breast cancer, you will too, or the notion that because hypertension runs in
your family you are destined to suffer a heart attack.

How can you stop your thoughts, feelings, and beliefs from inviting
illness into your life? How can you disable their destructive potential?
Essentially, this entails dismantling the architecture of your attitudes and
awareness of your body, your health, and illness. Although you can't erase
your mental surface like a chalkboard, you can lay down new mental
blueprints that cultivate wellness rather than illness. If your thoughts can
invite illness, they can also invite wholeness, joy, and reverence for life.
Adding just one such thought to our repertoire of mental images can melt
the misperceptions of illness that seem frozen into our unconscious just as
one light bulb can light up an entirely dark room. The benefits of this
approach, sometimes referred to as "cognitive restructuring," have been
validated by research on tens of thousands of patients suffering from a vast
array of diseases, including allergy, asthma, angina, arthritis, backache,
cancer, colitis, hypertension, migraine and many others.

Already, as you have been reading these pages, you have begun the hard but rewarding work of clearing space in your "mental garden" for new beliefs and interpretations of illness and medicine. As these thoughts grow, their roots will establish themselves deeply in the field of your mind, and once that happens, no illness-inducing thought will be able to shake them loose. "If you change your mind you change the world." So goes an ancient Zen Buddhist saying, echoing the same sentiment Jesus expressed when he proclaimed, "As you think, you are." The world you change when you transform your mental perceptions is the world within you. A change in your mental outlook unleashes a world of wellness within. The experience of wellness will register itself in every part of your body, flourishing there while new aspects of wellness unfold, like petals of a lotus blossom, in your soul.

THE PATIENT IS ALWAYS IN CHARGE

As you begin to change your role in your own health care, as you become a more active agent in the process of healing, the character and dimensions of the patient–physician relationship necessarily change as well. The new patient–physician relationship is more of a partnership for health, a collaboration in the process of healing. The new collaboration is based on both partners' shifting awareness of the other's role. For patients, this means accepting that there are limits to what a doctor can do for you and adjusting your expectations of your physician accordingly. For doctors, the new partnership requires recognizing, honoring, and respecting the intricate and mighty healing potential housed in the soul of every single patient and making the commitment to help patients recognize the same.

Risky Business

Patients possess the single most powerful instrument for healing. Nothing in my traditional doctor's bag nor in the entire Mayo Clinic can approach that depth. Seek out physicians who respect their patients as partners in the essentially spiritual pursuit of health. Never underestimate the magnitude of the awesome Healing Force that is within you. It is a process so stunning that the most advanced medical science can gather very little sense of what exactly is at work. And no medical procedure can replicate its complex and confounding expression. The Healing Force responds to a source higher than science, an *Omni-science*, or *Omniscience*.

This point was urged by the late editor of the *New England Journal of Medicine*, who cautioned his medical colleagues never to forget the power of their patients' own healing resources to remedy illness and disease. Rather than making doctors fearful that their skills may be required in fewer cases or concerned that unqualified practitioners will administer untested and potentially dangerous treatment therapies, the Healing Force now challenges all physicians to address the gaps in their training and in the excellent care they have been trained to provide.

Physicians must recognize that investing their patients with a greater sense of responsibility for health care does not diminish their own. Indeed, it sets in motion the healing process that the physician's treatment both enhances and is enhanced by. Some doctors worry that too little is known about the interplay of emotions, attitudes, ideas, and beliefs to imbue them with much meaning and prefer to stick instead to the physical symptoms that can be known. Yet doctors take risks all the time. Every time they prescribe a drug, doctors (and more important, their patients) risk the side effects that may accompany the drug. Every time a patient undergoes surgery, he or she is subjected to a number of risks that the physician weighs carefully before recommending the procedure. Risk taking is a central part of the processes of science and healing. It has been reliably estimated that somewhere between 80 and 90 percent of medical practices have not been evaluated as carefully as they should. In other words, presently, doctors have very little certainty about the consequences or results of the overwhelming majority of practices and procedures they rely on daily. Medicine, it seems, is risky business.

But why is it that physicians are willing to take risks with, and have more faith in, the science of technology and prescription drugs than the science of the soul and the body's own powerful Healing Force? Why are doctors often more ready to provide a powerful drug with dangerous side effects than to prescribe a large dose of hope, relaxation, forgiveness, or love? Why are we—patients and physicians—more likely to trust in the potential of a foreign substance or high-tech surgical procedure than we are to place our faith in our own natural healing resources?

Some of the answers to these tough questions have already been explored in this book. At this point it should be clear that our current medical system is built upon a passive patient–physician relationship. Like a machine, the patient is expected to passively accept the physician's input. This is not entirely the fault of physicians, who are but one level of a complex and competitive medical economy and who must respond to the constant demands from hospital administrators and insurance and pharmaceutical companies. Working under such pressures is enough to squelch any person's hopeful outlook, and indeed a good many physicians experience disillusionment before they finish with their training. But patients also play a role in this equation. Faced with illness, we tend to attach value to pills instead of valuing our selves and the underlying source of illness that is requesting our attention. Many of my patients have wanted to see me as little more than a pill fairy who can reach into my magic pocket and pull out a miracle drug.

Caring for your health should never be narrowly defined as a physical endeavor. Narrow definitions produce narrow results, and this book is about cultivating a total health—one that unfolds from the inner reaches of your soul and envelopes the entirety of your body, mind, and soul. It is never too late to learn to tend to the requirements of your mental and spiritual gardens, weeding out illness-inducing thoughts and emotions and replanting in their place the hopeful, soulful seeds of wellness that, when carefully nurtured, will become your harvest of health.

John Williams, the depressed patient who raised horses, came to see me about the profound problem he was experiencing and made it very clear that he was sick and tired of feeling like a walking side effect from all the antidepressant medication he had been taking. In his straightforward manner he told me why he believed he was depressed in the first place, and moreover, he was convinced that the depression he was suffering from was the result of all of the anger and frustration he had bottled up inside of him over the years.

From the very first moment he walked into my office, John Williams made it plain as day that he was willing to be a partner in his health care. He knew from experience that any treatment that lacked his personal involvement would be short-lived. Sitting across from me at my desk, he leaned close and waved a finger as he addressed me: "I want to explain to you that I am no doctor but I honestly feel that all the medicine that doctors have been giving me is like a paint job on an old car. It makes it look great on the outside, but it hasn't changed a thing on the inside."

Quick fixes may satisfy both patient and physician in the short term, but that satisfaction is only fleeting. In the long run, the soul still aches, and until that ache is addressed properly and with care from both physician and patient, all treatments will be temporary. Like a paint job on an old car.

Hope for Healing

The collaboration for healing between you and your doctor must be forged with hope. I am acutely sensitive to both physicians' and patients' concerns that in the face of a serious, perhaps life-threatening illness, too much hope may be misleading. Illness demands a sense of realism. But overcoming illness requires large doses of hope and in a collaborative effort for healing, physicians must encourage a feeling of hopefulness in their patients, particularly by making their own hopefulness visible.

Some physicians may argue that their responsibility is to present a reasonable picture of the patient's prognosis, without "doctoring" the hard facts. While I agree that doctors must always be honest with their patients and respect their need to know the likelihood for recovery, I also believe that doctors must be honest about the fact that much of what drives the recovery process we cannot medically explain. *Idiopathic Spontaneous Remission* is the term doctors use to account for what others might call "miracle cures," which basically means that something occurred that transcends any scientific logic and confounds even the best medical predictions. Never worry that you may have "false hope." That is an oxymoron! There is simply no such thing. Hope is never "false," because its origin is in the soul, the "best part" of you, the source of all truth.

There are no limitations to the healing process as long as the tissues or the organs involved are not dead. It is important that you take advantage of the best that medical science has to offer, but it is also important for you to be willing to take the responsibility to do whatever is personally necessary to help the healing process. Your health is much too important to be unscientific about; however, it is also much too important to leave up to science.

Soulful medicine is based on a new and dynamic collaboration for health that enables doctors and patients to engage the resources of hope and the wish to be well as much as they enlist the resources of drugs and surgery. The words spoken by Seneca more than two thousand years ago are just as relevant today: "It is part of the cure to wish to be cured."

HOW TO CREATE A PARTNERSHIP WITH YOUR DOCTOR

- Send your doctor a brief letter informing him or her of the active contribution you are now making to your health and well-being. Include a statement similar to this: "I realize that my health, in large measure, depends on the care I invest in myself as much as the expert care provided by you, my physician." (Note: if you are currently under your physician's care for any medical condition, this may be better handled in a personal consultation. Do not stop any medications without consulting your physician.)

- Include a copy of your signed Wellness Rx that outlines the promises you have made to yourself concerning your health. Ask your doctor to keep this copy in your medical records, and review it with him or her during your next office visit.

- Ask questions during your medical appointments. Do not be reluctant or embarrassed to inquire about results of tests, treatment procedures, or preventative measures. Remember, you have a right to this information and to discuss it with your physician. If your doctor seems in a hurry, it is okay to say, "Would you please spend a few more minutes discussing this with me. I cannot be an effective partner in my health care unless I am adequately informed."

- Be visibly interested and responsive. Keep the channels of communication flowing in both directions. It is not necessary to socialize. Ask direct questions and ask for specific answers. Remember that the typical physician will interrupt you after you have spoken for 18 seconds so keep your comments short.

- Always ask your doctor about responsible alternative treatments that are less invasive or less expensive. Always inquire about new developments in preventative care. Doctors will be much more likely to provide information on self-care and responsible alternatives if they know that you are willing to put in some personal effort. Keep in mind that most patients prefer a quick shot of medication over a strategy that requires greater responsibility over time. Let your doctor know that you are different.

- Expect excellent and expert care from your doctor, but be realistic. Remember, there are no magic bullets, and your doctor has no miracle cures. Sometimes when doctors sense that their patients are looking at them as superhuman, they react by being uncommunicative or dismissive. Respect your doctor's knowledge; however, don't expect him or her to know everything. Also, remember at all times that *M.D.* is not an abbreviation for "minor diety."

- Keep a health notebook containing your own record of your health, any symptoms or signs of discomfort. Note changes in your weight, skin tone, strength, and energy. Include information about your mental and spiritual energy too.

- Bring your notebook with you on any office visits and jot down important things that your doctor says so that you may refer back to them later. Tell your doctor you are keeping your own record and share it if you want to. Write down the questions you wish to have answered and write down the answers.

- If your doctor prescribes a drug for you, ask about the following: What is the drug being prescribed for? What are possible side effects? How frequent are the doses? How much will it cost? Is there a generic equivalent? Are you really sure it will not interact negatively with other current medications?

- Send your doctor copies of articles you may come across in the newspaper or other journals on exercise, spiritual health, nutrition, or other topics important to you. Your doctor is busy and may overlook helpful information in the press. Likewise, ask your doctor to keep you updated on recent medical research he or she may be aware of that would interest you.

- Finally, remember this: your doctor is a medical expert. But only you can become the expert of your mind and soul. Only you can reach into that vital source of healing and unleash its healing power.

How to Gain Experience

Nothing that I have said, nothing can compare to the power of experiencing firsthand the feeling of your soul's presence as it expands throughout your body during the simple process of prayerful meditation taught earlier in this book. By doing nothing more than quieting the mind, stilling the body, and calming the breath, you can coax the soul's Healing Force to announce its presence and render its healing influence.

The bridge between anticipating illness and knowing that *your "soul" purpose is to be well* is the bridge of *experience*. You may have had this experience before. It is the same as the peace we feel when our mind is still like a calm lake. It is the same as the satisfaction and joy we feel when we help someone else purely out of love. Soulful Medicine is about learning to turn that experience into an everyday occasion simply by increasing your awareness of the peace, joy, and love surrounding you and within you. In this book you have learned how to enhance and direct the natural healing process already occurring in your body—even without your awareness. The lessons in this book do not rely on "quick fixes." Soulful Medicine does, however, rely on the daily miracles of healing that are part of the body's natural state. The Wellness Rx is designed to help you unfold this natural state more fully from within so that you may experience a life of new and dynamic health and energy.

As I wrote near the beginning of this book, everybody—every ill, tired, stressed, diseased, depressed body—has the potential to be well. The first step on this bridge to wellness is the firm belief that health does not enter you from outside your body. Wellness, like all things sacred, emerges from deep within. To realize and experience this, you need to have some of the fearlessness of an infant learning to walk for the first time, and the humility of a child may also provide the key to reverence for life and soulful vitality. Fostering this fearlessness requires no daring feats, only faith and an effort on your part to think differently about your body, your health, and your beliefs. The Healing Force awaits.

EPILOGUE: HEALING OUT OF THE BLUE

Originally I planned to end this book with a discussion of how a new national health-care policy might be formulated around a vision of health care that addresses the whole person, not just physical symptoms, and that empowers individuals to assume responsibility for their own health destiny. But then I received a phone call that would reaffirm everything I believe about healing and nature and imbue those beliefs with a sense of immediacy, urgency, epiphany.

The call was from a young resident at a hospital in northern California, with whom I had had the privilege of working while he was still a medical student at the University of California, where I was on staff. He was the kind of young physician who reminds us veterans why we entered this profession—the ideals, the commitment, the eagerness to do good. David was calling for advice, as he occasionally did, but this time it was not about a patient or a diagnostic dilemma. He was calling to tell me about an experience on the Life Flight helicopter, an experience that made no medical sense to him but that nonetheless was etched in his memory as one of the most significant moments of his medical career.

David was to accompany a twenty-five-year-old man in an emergency situation during transport to a hospital in San Francisco for an urgent lung transplant. The patient had cystic fibrosis and had been in the intensive care unit of a Sacramento hospital for one month. Cystic fibrosis is a hereditary lung disease that causes the lungs to fill with thick fluid and to become infected. The patient was at the end stage of the disorder, the point when even a ventilator barely kept him breathing enough to survive.

When the physician in San Francisco called David to report that a lung was immediately available for transplant, the patient was suffering from a terrible pneumonia and was barely alive. Arrangements were quickly made to transport the patient by helicopter with the help of a portable breathing machine. His family was on the landing pad anxious and hopeful beneath a cloudy, rainy sky. It was raining so heavily there were doubts that the flight would go forth. David and several nurses tried to prepare the patient for the short but precarious flight. The portable breathing machine was not providing enough support. The medical team adjusted the settings, but the machine was not sophisticated or powerful enough to provide the oxygen the patient needed to survive. The oxygen in the patient's blood dropped even lower, and it was clear that hooked up to the portable machine he would not survive the ride.

The helicopter shut down its engine, and the patient's family grew visibly concerned. The threat of thundershowers remained, one more factor that might impede the mission. David and the nurses considered their limited options. A more powerful machine would be too big to fit into the helicopter. The only possibility of survival during transport was to breathe for the patient manually with a bag. David tested the procedure at the doors leading to the landing pad and determined that the manual pump would work adequately to give the patient enough oxygen to make the trip to San Francisco. Recognizing this might be their only chance to try, the team rushed the patient onto the helicopter.

The droning whirl of the helicopter propellers kicked into motion, and the emotional goodbyes from family members could barely be heard. Nearly ready to take off, David and the accompanying nurse were distressed to see that the patient's blood oxygen level had dropped frighteningly low again. Transport to San Francisco was looking less likely. They quickly suctioned out the fluid from the patient's lungs and administered medicine to keep the patient alive. Nothing was working. The blood oxygen level remained dangerously low.

David was seconds away from aborting the mission. He saw the whole family on the heliport praying, the nurse was praying, and David too began to pray that the patient would make it and that they could get him safely to San Francisco, where a transplant might save his life. Just as David was about to cancel the mission the patient's blood oxygen level elevated just high enough that the trip to San Francisco seemed manageable. After fifteen tense minutes on the landing pad, they were headed for San Francisco.

A MIRACLE IN THE SKY

David described the scene to me, calling it the tensest situation he'd ever been in. He was squeezing the bag and pumping oxygen into his patient's lungs. Stressed and anxious, he kept his mind on trying to maintain the patient's blood oxygen level at least as high as 90 percent to prevent permanent brain damage. Using everything in his physical power, David kept pumping and was just able to maintain the patient's blood oxygen level at 90 percent.

David looked away from his stiff and aching hands, pumping furiously, and focused on the deep murmur and hum of the helicopter. The sound carried his mind away, and he realized he was not thinking about his technique anymore. He was praying for his patient's life, that they would make it to San Francisco, that he would find the continued strength to keep the life in this man's lungs. He looked out the window, and all of a sudden, beneath a blanket of dark gray clouds, the sun appeared shining directly through the window of the helicopter. The cabin was illuminated in brilliant light. At this moment David realized that God was helping them out. He focused on that thought as he continued to look out the window, ignoring the monitor, still pumping but no longer concentrating on the technique or his tired hands. The nurse called out to him: "Doctor, it's 95 percent and holding steady!" It was the highest the patient's blood oxygen had been since they left the hospital. Filled with elation and hope, David bent over his patient and said, "You're going to make it." He kept his eyes out the window, watching the enormous ocean and the rhythm of the waves as they sped up the coast. When they landed in San Francisco he realized that without controlling his hands, they had been moving to the rhythm of the prayer he kept repeating over and over in his mind: "God, help this man live. God, help this man live."

A month later, David was asked to present this case at a conference before fifty other physicians. He was hesitant to describe the mission in much detail because there was nothing, in strict medical terms, very unusual about it. What was exciting, and what remained in David's mind as well as the nurse's, was the total feeling of God's presence in the helicopter on that tense ride to San Francisco. Nonetheless, he presented the medical facts of the case and described the technique he and the nurse employed to maintain the patient's blood oxygen level. As much as he fought back the urge to tell the whole story, David couldn't deny what really happened. And so he told the doctors the entire story. When he described the sun coming in through the helicopter window everyone burst into laughter. One doctor quipped, "Maybe the patient's body was more in tune with the compliance of his doctor's brain."

After the talk only the nurses approached David with serious comments, remarking how meaningful it was for them to hear a doctor acknowledge the powerful spiritual aspects of healing that nurses deal with so often. Some of the doctors approached him to find out what kind of drugs he—meaning, David—was on during the transport. But later in the week many of the doctors present at the talk cornered David one on one to tell him, "You know, I've had experiences like that too." One doctor told him, "You were brave to admit that in front of a bunch of doctors."

I suppose that David called me because he knew that I had long since determined never to be discouraged by physicians' general lack of faith in a healing power greater than our own or their disdain for any approach to medicine that embraces a spiritual dimension. Although the response of the doctors in David's audience did not surprise me—I've seen it many times before—I understood that for a young doctor with tremendous expertise such a reception was difficult to brush off at the beginning of his career. We talked it over for a long time, and by the end of our phone call, David recognized the laughter for what it was—nervousness. Nervousness and embarrassment in the face of the scientifically unexplainable.

A Trauma Turns into Triumph

"So what if your colleagues are only interested in learning about the scientific techniques relevant to the case. What did *you* learn from this experience?"

"I learned, in a way I was not prepared for, that anything is possible when you open your heart and mind to a higher healing power. Anything."

"You know, David, I have always believed that God's presence is behind all forms of healing. Your colleagues who are mostly interested in methods and procedures fail to recognize that there is something sacred about the healing process. In doing so, they limit the healing potential. When you looked out the window and experienced God's presence, you automatically enhanced your ability to help your patient heal."

"I also learned that our patients would probably benefit a great deal if we could spiritualize the practice of medicine even just a little bit."

"Yes, you are absolutely right. Medicine with a soul."

We hung up the phone, and I thought about how much I love this profession because of young doctors like David, men and women who bring to medicine a new appreciation of their patients' capacity to heal. I thought of the possibilities for medicine, Soulful Medicine, as we verge on the twenty-first century. While our nation's planners seek to define a new chapter in health care, I can't help but think that we might learn something from the ancient physicians who knew that it was as important to care for the soul as much as they cared for the body.

But do not wait for the others to carve out a new health-care system. The moment for you to take control of your own health destiny is now. What is there to stop you? Only yourself. You are the expert. And your own Healing Force is the most powerful healer of all. In this book I have tried to help you create the conditions in which your own inner physician can begin to take responsibility for your health destiny. Never underestimate your ability to heal. That is your nature.

A Word from Anneli Taub:

We have presented "Voyage to Wellness" programs on ships such as the *Queen Elizabeth II, Sagafjord, Stardancer, Niew Amsterdam, Caribe*, and *Windstar* on over fifty oceangoing journeys. The nighttime stars and endlessly rolling waves always provide a perfect setting to encourage and teach people to be more responsible for their health destiny. However, when it comes down to diet and nutrition, people always ask me "But what do you actually eat?"

This cookbook is the answer to that inevitable question. *This is what we actually eat.* During a recent month, we tested (and had great fun in the process!) all the recipes in this book. We ate these dishes for lunch or for dinner (the doctor recommends eating abundant quantities of fresh fruit for breakfast and *very* little else). The recipes are not always *very* low in fat, and the cookbook is not *entirely* vegetarian.

Sometimes, indeed, the cookbook gets downright decadent—especially the potato latkes, which are just an *occasional* holiday treat. But the underlying theme of the way *we* eat is that eating well doesn't require fanaticism or giving up fond memories and deep ethnic roots. I learned to cook while standing beside my mother as a very little girl growing up in Germany. My husband's taste buds were also shaped at a very early age by his Russian and Polish family.

I cook foods in a manner that makes the following recipes particularly savory—this is what we both remember. However, most of the eggs, milk, and cream, and all of the red meat we grew up with, are gone, and the fat content has been drastically slashed (believe me, more than 50 percent in each traditional recipe). We certainly don't eat junk food, we limit flesh food to about once a week, we never have red meat, and we virtually never eat anything with fat except during our main meal.

We are both *very* healthy and well. I am very slim, and my husband is just about the right weight with a tiny pot around his belly—which I happen to like, even though it discourages him a little bit. *Our cholesterol counts including HDL and LDL are excellent.*

These recipes are not based on science. They are based on taste, experience, tradition, and love—lots of each. If the good doctor had *his* own way, we would probably eat pasta five days a week for dinner and alternate that with matzoh brie, kasha varnishkes, potato pierogen, spinach and potatoes, or my vegetable soup with homemade bread.

I know that it's fat that makes us fat, and I am aspiring to be a true vegetarian, but I *still* like chicken because where I grew up it was such a treat. So we eat chicken about once a week (with the skin removed and the amount of canola oil used for frying reduced drastically). The one fish dish we occasionally eat is a salmon (or tuna) and pasta dish that is so good it is a cause for celebration. We *never* eat beef or pork.

Breakfasts at our house consist of abundant quantities of fresh fruit and fruit juice (we squeeze it), butterless bagels or homemade bread with fruit jam, occasional oatmeal or whole-grain cereal, and a cup of coffee or tea. No flesh, no fat.

My husband just grazes along until dinnertime, eating more fresh fruit, wholesome bread, fresh vegetables in salads or sandwiches, and occasionally a few nuts. In other words: no flesh, no fat.

Here we also share with you our new eating memories from our voyages throughout the world—adopted to the way we eat at home. Part of the enjoyment of traveling comes from experiencing the varied dining delights of other cultures, and part of the joy of returning home is sharing such experiences with family and friends. A quote comes to mind attributed to Zorba the Greek from someone who had painted it on the ceiling of an old country inn we visited for lunch in the Corsican highlands: "I have decided after all, that good dining is a spiritual experience!"

A Husbandly Note:

Before there was counting calories, there were people who were thin. Before there was counting grams of fat, there were people without coronary artery disease. Anneli steadfastly refuses to count either calories or grams of fat but slashes the quantities of both while still providing dishes that would still make all of our grandmothers smile if they were alive. This cookbook is a month's worth of what we actually eat. We have one main meal of the day and then "graze" along the rest of the time without fat or flesh. I have never eaten as well and as healthfully in all my life. *Buon appetito!*

APPENDIX:
RECIPES FROM
ANNELI'S GARDEN
OF EATING

Salads

Anneli's Fast Green Bean Salat
Fresh Tomato Salad
Swabian Cucumber Salat
Caesar's Salat à la Laguna
Potato and Cucumber Salat

Appetizers & Dips

Sue's Roasted Garlic
Spicy Peanut Dip
Tzatziki Dip

Soups, Breads, & Sandwiches

Orange Carrot Caribbean Soup
Broccoli Creme Soup
Mama's Green Bean Soup
Black Forest Bread
Scones
The St. John's Island Special
Quesadilla Suprema

Pasta

Pasta Guiseppe
Pasta Primavera Surpriso
Pasta Camembert
Lasagna Verdura
Artichoke Heart-Angel Hair
Penne All'Arrabbiata (Almost!)
Pasta Alta Cunard
Stuffed Shells
Corzetti à la Rivieresca

Vegetables & Cheese

Ratatouille Provencal
Vegetable Wellington
Feta à la Grecque
Thai Tofu Satay

Chicken

Chicken Tarragon with Couscous
Chicken Fricassée a la Berlin
Hunter Chicken Goulash
Pollo All'Arrabbiata

Old World Delights

Kasha Varnishkes
Potato Pancakes Eleonore
Potato Pirogen
Matzoh Brie
Spinach and Mashed Potatoes

HELPFUL HINTS AND COOKING TIPS

- For my sautéing and frying needs I use high quality nonstick cookware.
- Maggi is a wonderful addition to hearty soups and flavorful recipes. You will find it in health-food stores. If you can't get Maggi, tamari sauce or bragg can be substituted.
- A salad spinner–dryer is a great investment to achieve wonderful green salads.
- IMPORTANT! Always taste your cooking. Recipes are always subjective. Trust your taste. Be inventive!
- Don't skimp on buying the very best olive oil. Purchase organic cold-pressed extra-virgin olive oil. Products that are just labelled "pure" or "virgin" are inferior.

Anneli's Fast
Green Bean Salat

A delicious, quick, and simple bean salad. The unusual combination of pepper, sugar, and Maggi makes this dish irresistible. Look for Maggi in the gourmet foods section at your market or at a local gourmet foods store. A terrific side dish to complement pierogies or matzoh brie.

Serves 2.

1 14 oz. can French-cut green beans, drained
1 Tbsp. onion, finely grated
1 Tbsp. vinegar
¼ tsp. salt
1 tsp. Maggi
Dash each of pepper and sugar
1 Tbsp. canola oil

Drain the water from the beans and empty them into a bowl. Add all the ingredients and mix well so that all of the beans are soaked with dressing. If you like, garnish with chopped fresh parsley.

Fresh Tomato Salad

Fresh, sweet Roma tomatoes are essential to this cool salad. Because it's light, it can be served with cheese and bread for lunch, or as a side dish for dinner. A delicious complement to Artichoke Heart–Angel Hair pasta.

Serves 2.

5 ripe Roma tomatoes, sliced
1 tsp. onion, finely grated
¼ tsp. salt
½ tsp. sugar
Dash pepper
2 Tbsp. vinegar
½ Tbsp. parsley, finely chopped
½ tsp. Maggi, available in gourmet sections
1 Tbsp. canola oil

Place sliced tomatoes in a bowl and add the onions, seasonings, and oil. Mix well to cover tomatoes evenly. Serve immediately.

Swabian Cucumber Salat

Cool, crisp, and delicious!

Serves 2.

1 large cucumber, peeled
½ Tbsp. small onion, grated very finely
1½ Tbsp. white vinegar
½ tsp. sugar
½ tsp. salt
½ tsp. Maggi
2 tsp. canola oil

Slice the peeled cucumber *very thin* and place in a bowl. Add remaining ingredients and combine well.

Caesar's Salat à la Laguna

A local variation on a long-standing classic! We've left out the egg for lighter texture and lower fat. Creative and flavorful, this robust salad can be served as the main dish itself, which is how we like to eat it, with a crunchy loaf of French bread.

Serves 4.

1 small bunch Romaine lettuce, washed and cut in 2-inch pieces
2 cloves garlic, minced*
1 inch anchovy paste, or 1 anchovy fillet, mashed
½ Tbsp. Dijon mustard
½ Tbsp. Worcestershire sauce
Juice of ½ lemon
¼ tsp. pepper
2 Tbsp. olive oil
3 Tbsp. Parmesan cheese, grated

In a medium-sized bowl mash garlic together with anchovy. Add mustard, Worcestershire sauce, lemon juice, pepper, and olive oil. Whisk until creamy, then add the Parmesan cheese and mix. Add lettuce and toss well.

*If you are not a great garlic lover, instead of mashing 2 cloves, slice 1 clove in half, exposing its juices, and rub it over the inside of your bowl. This technique works best with a wooden bowl and leaves just enough hint of garlic.

Potato and Cucumber Salat

This cool and tangy salad is lighter than most potato salads and is terrific on a warm day for lunch or with Hunter Chicken Goulash for dinner.

Serves 4.

4 medium red potatoes
½ small onion, grated very finely
½ cucumber, peeled and grated
1 tsp. salt
½ tsp. pepper
1 tsp. Maggi
1 tsp. sugar
3 Tbsp. vinegar
2 Tbsp. canola oil

Boil potatoes about 30 minutes until soft. Let stand in cold water for 5 minutes. (This makes peeling easier.) Then peel and cool in a medium-sized bowl. Slice cooled potatoes *very* finely. Then grate peeled cucumber and onion very finely. Continue with the rest of the ingredients. Mix well.

NOTE: If too dry, use a bit of warm water to obtain smooth consistency.

Sue's Roasted Garlic

If you like garlic, or even if you don't, you'll love this dish as an appetizer. We were skeptical when our good friend and excellent chef Sue placed this aromatic dish in front of us, but one taste totally turned our minds around. Because it is baked slowly, the garlic becomes creamy like a soft spread, baking out all of the strong flavor we associate with fresh garlic. Serve with plenty of good French bread.

Serves 4.

4 heads garlic (large buds are best)
Salt and pepper
1 Tbsp. olive oil

Preheat oven to 275°. Peel away the outer skin of the garlic heads and use a sharp knife to flatten out the base so that the garlic will sit upright (pointed end up). Place garlic in a small baking dish. Add a few shakes of salt and pepper and bake.

After 30 minutes, remove the garlic from the oven and sprinkle a little olive oil over each head. Return garlic to oven for one more hour. The garlic is done when the buds separate easily from the heads.

Serve tepid, squeezing each bud from its skin directly onto bread and spreading with a knife.

Spicy Peanut Dip

This exotic mixture is just right for dipping raw vegetables like carrots, celery, cauliflower, broccoli, and zucchini. Or try it spread on pita bread.

Serves 4.

2 Tbsp. canola oil
1 small onion, finely chopped
2 cloves garlic, crushed
¼ tsp. chili powder
1 tsp. ground cumin
1 tsp. ground coriander
6 Tbsp. crunchy peanut butter (no sugar added)
4 oz. water
1 tsp. lemon juice
1 tsp. soy sauce

Heat the oil in a pan and fry onions until soft. Add garlic and spices and stir for 1 minute. Mix in the peanut butter and gradually add water, blending until thick. Add lemon juice and soy sauce and remove from heat. Let cool thoroughly before serving.

Tzatziki Dip

*Great for dipping raw vege-
tables or spreading on fresh
pita bread.*

Serves 2.

1 cup plain low-fat yogurt
1 garlic clove, crushed
1 Tbsp. fresh mint, chopped
½ tsp. salt
½ tsp. pepper
1 small cucumber, peeled, seeded, and
  grated

Empty yogurt into a bowl, add garlic, salt,
pepper, and mint. Stir in grated cucumber
and combine ingredients well.

Orange Carrot
Caribbean Soup

*Friends in the South Carib-
bean made us this soup for
the first time. The warm
spices and sweet carrots are
a wonderful combination for
warm or cold weather.
Serve with a fresh baguette.*

Serves 2.

½ Tbsp. butter
1 tsp. curry powder
6 carrots, cleaned and cut into ¼-inch
  slices
1 large orange
2 tsp. lemon juice
1 cup water
1 tsp. salt
½ tsp. pepper
2 Tbsp. cilantro, chopped
½ tsp. sugar

Slice the orange in half and squeeze its
juice, including the pulp. Keep the peel of
one half and shave into thin twists.

In a skillet melt the butter and add curry,
leaving on low heat for 5 minutes while stirring to bring out the flavor of the curry.
Add carrots and stir for 8 minutes. Add orange juice, and pulp. Next, add water, lemon
juice, salt, pepper, and sugar. Cook for 20
minutes on medium heat until carrots are
tender, then cover.

Transfer ingredients to a blender and puree
to a smooth consistency. Return soup to skillet and reheat. Serve garnished with orange
twists and chopped cilantro.

Broccoli Creme Soup

Thick and creamy, this soup is perfect for a cold night and is incredibly easy to prepare.

Serves 2.

1 medium onion, chopped
5 small stems broccoli, florets and stems
½ Tbsp. canola oil
1 cup water
¼ cup half-and-half
1½ tsp. salt
Dash pepper
1 cup walnuts, chopped

Wash and peel broccoli. Chop stems and florets into small pieces. Heat oil and sauté onion for 10 minutes. Add broccoli pieces and sauté for 10 minutes. Add water and cook covered on low heat for 30 minutes. Let cool and transfer to blender. Puree until very fine. Return soup to pot and add half-and-half, salt, and pepper. Keep warm. In another pan, lightly toast the chopped walnuts for 10 minutes, stirring frequently. Add to soup and serve hot.

Mama's Green Bean Soup

Fresh green beans are the secret to this hearty, robust soup. If fresh beans are not available, frozen is the next best thing. This is a good recipe to make if there are children in the house—they love the sound of popping off the ends and breaking the beans in half!

Serves 4.

3 cups green beans, remove ends and break in half
5 cups water
2 Tbsp. summer savory herb
2½ Tbsp. canola oil (½ Tbsp. for browning onions; 2 Tbsp. for browning flour)
2 medium onions, finely chopped
3 Tbsp. Wondra® flour
2 tsp. salt
1 Tbsp. sugar
2 Tbsp. vinegar
1 lb. wide egg noodles

Boil water and summer savory. Add beans to boiling water and cook for 20 minutes.

While beans cook, heat ½ Tbsp. canola oil and sauté onions until brown. In a small skillet, heat 2 Tbsp. canola oil and add flour, stirring constantly so it won't clump, until it smokes and looks brown.

Add the onions and flour to the beans and stir. Add vinegar, salt, and sugar, and let simmer for 10 minutes.

While soup simmers, boil water for noodles and cook noodles until al dente. Serve soup hot, over the noodles.

Black Forest Bread

You don't need a bread machine to enjoy this tasty, healthful bread. This family recipe originates in Germany and has remained a favorite for the last three generations. It is espcially easy to make if you have a mixer with dough hooks.

4 cups unbleached white flour or bread flour
2 cups rye flour
1 4-oz. packet rapid-rise yeast
½ Tbsp. salt
7 oz. buttermilk, or plain nonfat yogurt
8 oz. warm water
½ medium raw potato, finely grated
1 Tbsp. cornmeal

Important! All ingredients should be room temperature.

Mix the flours and salt together. Sprinkle in the yeast and add the warm water, potato, and buttermilk (or yogurt). Knead with an electric mixer using dough hooks for 10 minutes or by hand for 20 minutes. Knead until dough no longer sticks to your hands and the bowl. Cover with a towel and leave to rise in a warm place (on top of an oven set at 300° works well). Let rise until double in size, then punch it down. Shape into a round ball. Set the dough on a nonstick baking sheet, sprinkle with cornmeal, and poke one-inch deep holes all over the dough with a fork. Sprinkle the top with flour. Drape again with the towel to let rise for another 30 minutes on top of stove.

Fill an ovenproof casserole dish halfway with water and place on the lowest shelf in the oven. Preheat oven to 425°.

Now place dough on sheet in oven. Immediately lower heat to 375° and bake for 45 minutes or until brown crust develops. Bread is done when it makes a hollow sound when you knock on the bottom of the loaf.

Scones

Scones have made quite a comeback in the United States in the last few years. There's no end to the variety of scone you can make, flavored with everything from fruit to herbs. Here's a breakfast version that is simple to prepare and sure to be a favorite. A healthful alternative to high-fat donuts and muffins. We use raisins but have had success with blueberries, raspberries, mashed bananas, and cherries.

Makes 6 scones.

1 cup plain nonfat yogurt
1 egg
3 Tbsp. honey
3 cups unbleached flour
2 tsp. baking powder
1 tsp. baking soda
½ tsp. salt
⅓ cup melted butter
½ cup raisins
1½ tsp. grated orange peel

Preheat oven to 400°. Use a nonstick spray to cover a baking sheet.

Beat together yogurt, egg, and honey in a large bowl. In a separate bowl sift together flour, baking soda, baking powder, and salt. Stir two-thirds of the flour mixture into the wet ingredients and mix well. Add the melted butter. Stir in raisins, orange peel and remaining flour mix. Mix with a wooden spoon until stiff. Turn onto a lightly floured surface and knead gently, *only 3 or 4 times.* Too much kneading will result in a smooth surface, and scones should be lumpy on top. Divide dough into 6 pieces and place on baking sheet. Bake for 15 to 20 minutes, until golden brown.

If you use fresh fruit, fold it into dough very carefully. Many times I have stirred too vigorously and ended up with a blue scone!

The St. John's Island Special

On a sailboat headed for Catalina Island, eating these sandwiches with close friends, we closed our eyes and imagined we were sailing toward the Caribbean Island of St. John's. It was there that I was inspired by a local secret, safe off the well-trodden tourist path: the most unique honey mustard I have ever come across. I sat under a palm umbrella just beside the shacklike restaurant, aware of the creator's satisfied Caribbean grin as he watched me devour the best thing I'd eaten in weeks. He offered me a napkin to wipe away the sacred ingredient; I offer you the recipe he proudly imparted to me.

Serves 2–4.

The Mustard:
Combine a small jar of Dijon mustard with half that amount of honey. Dilute with the juice of a whole fresh lemon and stir.

The Sandwich:
Slice open a loaf of crusty Italian or French bread and spread the honey mustard very liberally over the inside. Line the bread with layers of each of the following fresh vegetables:

Sliced avocado
Sliced Roma tomatoes
Alfalfa sprouts
Sliced cucumber
Crisp lettuce
(Experiment with different vegetables, carrots, mushrooms, etc.!)

Top the vegetables with a thin layer of fresh cheese. Low-fat cheddar, Brie or even cream cheese tastes wonderful with the honey mustard.

Drizzle more honey mustard over the top of the sandwich filling, then close bread, slice, and, as the St. John's locals say, "Go to it, Man!"

Quesadilla Suprema

This Mexican dish is not really a "sandwich" but shares some of the same qualities. Still, it should be enjoyed in its authentic form, with fresh and spicy salsa and guacamole. Eat it whole or slice it into wedges, as an appetizer or as a meal in itself. Although the dips can be purchased already prepared at the market, take the extra time to make them from fresh ingredients yourself—the small effort will bring big rewards. Make a little extra for dipping blue or yellow corn chips.

Serves 2–4.

Guacamole:
Mix together
2 medium avocados
½ small onion, grated
Juice of ½ small lemon
1 tsp. Maggi (available in gourmet sections)

Salsa:
Mix together
5 medium tomatoes (Roma if available), diced
4 green onions, chopped
2 Tbsp. fresh cilantro, finely chopped
Juice of ½ small lemon
⅛ tsp. salt
1 small chili pepper, chopped (optional)

Quesadilla:
4 medium flour tortillas
1 Tbsp. canola oil
4 oz. lowfat cheddar or jack cheese, grated
4 oz. part-skim mozzarella, grated

Heat the oil in a medium-sized frying pan. Place a tortilla in the pan and cover with grated cheeses. Cover with another tortilla. Turn occasionally and cook over medium heat until golden brown. Drain on a paper towel to remove excess oil.

Serve hot with guacamole and salsa.

Pasta Guiseppe

This dish is dedicated to our dear friend Guiseppe, who was our maître d' during a long cruise. Guiseppe takes great pride in discovering the tiny details of his guests' "tastes" to help them enjoy their dining on ship. When he found out we were vegetarians (and the ship's doctor!), Guiseppe arranged this dish with the chef as a special surprise. It was one of our favorites, and we still enjoy it at home, with a delicious Caesar's Salad à la Laguna.

Serves 2.

2½ Tbsp. olive oil
6 cloves garlic
3 anchovy fillets, mashed, or 2 inches anchovy paste with ½ tsp. salt
¼ tsp. crushed red pepper
1 handful of fresh parsley, chopped
1 Tbsp. Parmesan cheese
½ lb. rigatoni

Boil water for pasta.

Peel and mash 3 garlic cloves and mix with anchovies. Add chopped parsley and pepper. Add 2 Tbsp. olive oil and stir until mixture resembles a creamy paste.

Add pasta to boiling water and cook until al dente.

Peel and slice remaining 3 garlic cloves and sauté in ½ Tbsp. olive oil until golden but not brown, about 1 minute.

Strain pasta and mix together well with the paste and sautéed garlic. Top with grated Parmesan cheese.

Pasta Primavera Surpriso

Pasta is a favorite in our cooking. This inexpensive grain comes in so many shapes and colors, made from a variety of sources. Fresh or dried, pasta is simple to cook and be creative with. This sauce is filled with fresh vegetables and seasonings, and the apricots give it an unusual twist.

Serves 2.

1½ Tbsp. olive oil
4 garlic cloves, sliced
10 mushrooms, sliced
4 medium-sized tomatoes (Roma if available), cubed
1 zucchini, sliced
2 carrots, sliced
2 apricots (dried is fine) or 1 small peach, cut in small pieces
¼ cup white wine
1 tsp. sugar
½ tsp. salt
1 pinch pepper
1 tsp. Italian herbs

Heat the olive oil in a large frying pan and add the sliced mushrooms. Stir constantly until the mushrooms become tender, then add the garlic. Stir in the zucchini, carrots, and apricots. Add wine and cook covered over low heat for 15 minutes. Add sugar, herbs, salt and pepper. Stir in the cubed tomatoes and cook for another 5 minutes. Add a little water if too dry.

Serve over hot linguini, artichoke-spinach spaghetti, or whole-wheat pasta and sprinkle with grated Parmesan cheese.

Pasta Camembert

Camembert cheese is so ripe and smooth it just soaks up the flavors of the herbs and spices in this dish and melts so easily over hot pasta. This recipe is a slight variation on a dish we first encountered in a tiny restaurant on the island of Elba in a town named Portefarraio. For a lighter version, substitute low-fat large-curd ricotta cheese.

Serves 2 with leftovers.

3 large sun ripened tomatoes, cut in small cubes
4 oz. Camembert cheese (or lowfat large-curd ricotta)
½ cup fresh basil, chopped, or Italian parsley if basil is unavailable
1 clove garlic, pressed
1½ Tbsp. extra virgin olive oil
1 tsp. salt
dash ground pepper
dash sugar
1 lb. pasta
grated fresh Romano cheese

Remove the rind from the Camembert cheese and break cheese into ½-inch cubes. In a large bowl, add the cheese and all ingredients except salt, pasta and Romano cheese. Let stand at room temperature for approximately 2 hours. Add salt.

Boil water and cook pasta to al dente. Drain pasta and quickly mix with cold ingredients. Serve immediately on warmed plates, topped with grated Romano cheese.

Lasagne Verdura

A rich and savory version of an old favorite! We've added lots of fresh mushrooms and substituted nonfat ricotta for the higher-fat variety. This lasagne is especially flavorful the next day.

Serves 6.

Sauce:
1 Tbsp. olive oil
3 cloves garlic, mashed
1 Tbsp. onions, finely chopped
4 cups mushrooms, sliced
2 large cans of tomatoes, whole, peeled
1 tsp. Italian herbs
1 tsp. sugar
½ tsp. salt
1 dash pepper
1 bay leaf

Heat the olive oil in a large pan; add the garlic, onions, mushrooms, and herbs; and stir until golden brown. In a large pot, empty the cans of tomatoes, mash, and then add the sugar, salt, pepper, and bay leaf. Stir in the onion and mushroom mixture. Cook on low heat for 20 minutes.

Ingredients:
15 wide lasagna noodles
3 bunches fresh spinach, or 2 packages frozen spinach
1 lb. mushrooms, washed and dried
30 oz. nonfat ricotta cheese

1 cup fresh parsley, chopped
2 medium onions, chopped
2 Tbsp. canola oil
1 cup Parmesan cheese, grated
3 cups grated lowfat mozzarella
1 egg
Salt

Boil a large pot of water with 1 Tbsp. canola oil and add the lasagna noodles to boiling water. Stir noodles and cook for 10 minutes, strain, and rinse with cold water. Separate to prevent sticking and set aside.

While pasta cooks, sauté mushrooms in ½ Tbsp. canola oil until all liquid has evaporated and mushrooms are brown, stirring often. In a separate skillet, sauté onions in ½ Tbsp. canola oil until brown.

Boil 2 cups of water and cook the spinach (if using fresh) for 10 minutes until reduced. Drain spinach and transfer to blender. Puree until very smooth. Sprinkle with 1 tsp. salt.

In a bowl, mix ricotta cheese with egg, 1 Tbsp. salt, chopped parsley, and Parmesan cheese.

Coat the bottom of a 9 × 13-inch casserole dish with 2 cups of the tomato sauce. Layer the ingredients in the following order: noodles, a thin layer of ricotta mixture, and all of the mushrooms. Add another layer of noodles, all of the spinach, half of the mozzarella, and all of the onions. Add another layer of noodles, the rest of the ricotta, a final layer of noodles, and 1 cup of tomato sauce, and sprinkle with Parmesan cheese. Cover with aluminum foil and bake at 350° for 40 minutes. Let stand 5 minutes before cutting. Serve with remaining tomato sauce.

Artichoke Heart–Angel Hair

The delicate texture of angel hair pasta in combination with the lively flavor of artichoke hearts make this dish, well, simply put . . . heavenly! Taking the extra time to prepare fresh artichokes is well worth the effort. If you do use canned, be certain to get hearts in water, not in oil, which will ruin this remarkably light dish. Serve with Fresh Tomato Salad and, of course, a good Italian bread.

Serves 2.

2 Tbsp. olive oil
1 small onion, finely chopped
1 clove garlic, mashed
10 medium mushrooms, sliced
⅓ cup slivered almonds
6 artichoke hearts, fresh or canned in
    water
1 large tomato, cubed
¼ tsp. salt
1 pinch of each: pepper, sugar, tarragon
⅓ cup wine
⅓ cup water
½ lb. angel hair pasta

Boil water for pasta.

In a large skillet, sauté the onion, garlic, mushrooms, and almonds in oil until slightly golden. Add the artichoke hearts, tomatoes, salt, pepper, sugar, and tarragon. Then add white wine and water and let simmer for 10 minutes.

While sauce simmers, cook pasta in boiling water for 8 minutes, until al dente.

If you choose to take the extra time to use fresh artichokes, prepare them in salted, boiling water for 40 minutes, or until a leaf pulls easily off. Remove all the leaves and surroundings of the heart and discard the straw around it. Save the leaves and eat them later with Tzatziki Dip.

Penne All'Arrabbiata (Almost!)

In Italian, arrabbiata *means "furious," which is no exaggeration considering how hot this dish is traditionally prepared all over Italy. We've toned it down a few degrees, but you can easily add more red pepper if you prefer the "furious" version!*

Serves 4.

2 tsp. olive oil
1 medium onion, chopped
4 garlic cloves, sliced
2 28-oz. cans tomatoes, peeled
¼ tsp. crushed red pepper (vary according to taste)
¼ tsp. Italian herbs
¼ tsp. salt
½ tsp. sugar
¼ tsp. pepper
8 pieces dried tomatoes cut into small pieces
1 lb. pasta
Parmesan cheese, grated

Sauté onion and garlic in oil over medium heat until just soft and glassy. Add tomatoes in their liquid, removing hard stems and breaking tomatoes into small pieces with a large spoon. Add crushed pepper, herbs, pepper, sugar, and salt to taste. Add dried tomatoes and simmer on medium heat for about 45 minutes, uncovered. Mash the sauce to medium consistency.

While sauce simmers, boil water for pasta and cook al dente. Drain and rinse pasta and serve covered hot with sauce and sprinkled with Parmesan cheese.

Pasta Alta Cunard

*Credit for this rich and delectable recipe goes to Chef Paul at the Alta Lodge in Utah. Die-hard skiers return from what are arguably the toughest slopes in the United States starved and in need of nourishment to re-energize them for another day of skiing. The only thing this bunch takes more seriously than skiing, maybe, is their dining. The culinary staff at Alta rivals the kitchens of the finest ski resorts in Europe, with a distinctly mountain spirit all their own. Away from the slopes and craving this dish, I improvised with the chef onboard the equally notorious **QE II**. Here is the best from the snow and the sea!*

Serves 4.

1 Tbsp. canola oil
1 medium carrot, thinly sliced
2 green onions, sliced (including tops)
1 medium zucchini, sliced
1 4-oz. can green peas, drained
1 8-oz. can asparagus pieces including
    liquid
1 tsp. fresh basil, chopped, or ½ tsp. dried
½ tsp. salt
Dash of white pepper and ground nutmeg
½ cup half-and-half
¼ cup Parmesan cheese
1 lb. spaghetti

Boil water for pasta.

Sauté in oil all of the vegetables except the peas and asparagus. Stir and simmer for 10 minutes. Add salt, pepper, basil, and nutmeg, then add half-and-half and Parmesan cheese. Stir carefully and simmer for 5 minutes. Add asparagus and peas, simmer for 10 more minutes.

While sauce simmers, cook pasta until al dente, drain, and rinse.

Serve sauce hot over spaghetti.

Stuffed Shells

These shells are a favorite amongst our beachtown friends. The thick and flavorful sauce keeps the cheese and pasta moist. Double the sauce recipe and store some away in the freezer for Lasagne Verdura to be made later. Serve with the easy and fast Fresh Tomato Salad.

Serves 4.

Prepare the tomato sauce following the recipe for Lasagne Verdura.

18 jumbo pasta shells

Filling:
1 package creamed spinach, frozen (prepare according to package instructions)
15 oz. nonfat ricotta cheese
1 cup Parmesan cheese, grated
1 small onion, finely chopped
1 clove garlic, mashed
1 egg white
2 tsp. salt
1 tsp. pepper

While the tomato sauce simmers, cook the pasta shells in boiling water until just soft, about 5 minutes. Drain and rinse with cool water, and separate to prevent from sticking.

Combine in a large bowl all of the ingredients for the filling. Stir well.

Pour a thin layer of tomato sauce in a 9 × 13-inch casserole dish. Stuff shells with filling and arrange, open side up, in the dish. Cover the filled shells with the remaining tomato sauce and bake, covered with foil, at 375° for 40 minutes.

Ratatouille Provencal

This fragrant blend of vegetables and spices fills our
kitchen with a scent like no
other dish! We like to eat it
hot, over rice. The next day
we enjoy the leftovers served
cold sprinkled with a little
fresh lemon juice.

Serves 4 (or 2 with
leftovers!).

2 garlic cloves, thinly sliced
2 medium onions, thinly sliced
1 Tbsp. olive oil
4 medium fresh tomatoes, 7 Roma toma-
    toes, or 1 8-oz. can whole tomatoes, cut
    into pieces
2 medium zucchini, cut into ¼-inch slices
1 small eggplant, cut into 1-inch pieces
1 medium bell pepper, sliced
1 tsp. herbs de Provence
½ tsp. each salt and pepper
1 Tbsp. lemon juice
Dash sugar

Heat oil and sauté onions and garlic until
glassy. Add tomatoes and simmer for 10 minutes, stirring frequently. Add remaining vegetables, herbs, and seasonings. Cover and
simmer on low heat for 30 minutes. Serve
steaming hot over rice.

Vegetable Wellington

We were greeted with this meatless variation on a culinary classic by the chef onboard a cruise ship traveling through the Caribbean Islands. The passengers seated with us, always amazed at our ability to pass up the fine gourmet meat dishes, were surprised at how decadent something so healthful could be. The next night they asked the waiter to bring them whatever the Doctor was having! Try not to think of this as a substitution for a meat dish—the natural flavors of the fresh vegetables are worthy of their own praise.

Fresh Tomato Tarragon Sauce:
2 tsp. olive oil
3 shallots, diced
1 clove garlic, minced
5 ripe tomatoes, peeled and diced
1 tsp. tarragon
¼ tsp. brown sugar
Salt and pepper to taste

Sauté the shallots and garlic in oil for 2 minutes. Add the tomatoes, tarragon, brown sugar, salt, and pepper. Simmer for 20 minutes, then mix lightly in the blender.

Wellington:
1 Tbsp. olive oil
2 small onions, finely chopped
1 garlic clove, finely diced
½ cup broccoli florets
½ cup mushrooms, sliced
¼ cup yellow squash, sliced thin lengthwise with seeds removed
1 Tbsp. parsley, chopped
Salt and pepper to taste
2 6-inch squares of puff pastry
1 egg white
1 Tbsp. nonfat milk

Sauté the onions, garlic, broccoli, mushrooms, squash, in olive oil. Add the parsley. Stir in half of the Fresh Tomato Tarragon Sauce.

Pour half of the mixture in the center of each pastry, fold up sides, and seal edges with part of the mixture of the egg white beaten with milk. Place the pastries on a cookie sheet with folded edges down and brush the top with remaining egg–milk mixture. Bake at 400° for 12 to 15 minutes or until brown. Cover pastry with the remaining sauce and serve immediately.

Corzetti à la Rivieresca

Common throughout the
southern regions of Europe,
this savory dish is truly
healthful. Filled with salmon
and walnuts, this main dish
provides a bounty of pro-
tein. The spiral-shaped pasta
and the shades of orange
and green make this dish as
beautiful to look at as it is
delightful to eat. If salmon
is not available, substitute
tuna canned in water (2 12-
oz. cans). Serve with a fresh
Ceasar's Salat.

Serves 4.

½ lb. fresh salmon filet, sliced and cut into
    small pieces (If unavailable use one 12½-
    ounce can of salmon in spring water)
1 tsp. canola oil
1 medium onion, finely chopped
2 cloves garlic, sliced thin
½ cup white wine
½ cup water
1 small can tomato paste
1 tsp. herbs de Provence
¾ cup walnuts, very finely chopped
Juice of one small lemon
1 tsp. sugar
Salt and pepper, to taste
1 lb. corzetti pasta (spirals)

Heat the oil and add the onions and garlic.
Sauté for 5 minutes or until the onions are
glassy. Add the salmon and white wine and
let simmer for 10 minutes. Stir constantly.
Add the tomato paste and ½ cup water, although consistency should not be too thin.
Add the herbs, sugar, salt, pepper, lemon
juice and walnuts. Simmer over low heat for
about 20 minutes, stirring constantly.

Serve hot over corzetti pasta.

Feta à la Grecque

This dish was unexpectedly discovered in a small German village. At home this is one of our newfound favorites. Those who have tried it insist that it be served as a main dish rather than simply an appetizer. The harmonious blend of spices do much to enhance the characteristically tangy taste of feta. Serve it with black olives and a crusty baguette for soaking up the flavorful sauce.

Serves 2.

Many's the long night I've dreamed of cheese—toasted, mostly.
    —Robert Louis Stevenson

Cut two 1-inch slices of Greek or domestic feta cheese. Line a piece of aluminum foil (big enough to wrap cheese in) with a piece of plastic wrap the same size. Place 1 slice of feta in the center of wrapping. Repeat for the second slice of feta.

Rub the feta generously all over with the following:
    2 Tbsp. paprika
    1 Tbsp. oregano
    garlic (about 2 cloves, mashed)

Then drizzle a few drops of olive oil over each slice. Fold foil neatly around feta, not too tight.

Heat oven to 350° and bake for 25 to 30 minutes. The plastic wrap will not melt. Serve hot out of the oven, atop a leaf of colorful lettuce.

Thai Tofu Satay

This dish is spicy and stimulating, like much of Thai food, although not quite as hot as some! It is not for the quiet or the shy, but rather this dish should be shared with a gathering of friends or family. We always make this dish for social occasions—it inspires conversation! Serve with Cucumber Salat.

Serves 4.

1 lb. tofu, extra firm, drained well and cut into ½-inch slices

Place tofu on a cookie sheet and bake in a 350° oven for 15 minutes; flip tofu and cook for another 10 minutes.

2 cloves garlic, mashed
½ Tbsp. vinegar
½ cup peanut butter
½ tsp. fresh ginger root, grated
2 Tbsp. honey
¼ cup soy sauce
¼ cup boiling water
½ tsp. salt
⅛ tsp. cayenne pepper (or slightly less chili powder)
1 Tbsp. cranberry sauce

Mix together all of the ingredients except the tofu. Pour three-fourths of the marinade into a 9 × 13-inch casserole dish. Place the baked tofu in a single layer in the pan and cover with the remaining sauce. Marinate for 2 hours. Bake at 375° for 25 minutes.

Serve hot over basmati rice.

For firm tofu, it is essential to bake it in slices on a greased cookie sheet for 15 minutes. This will create a golden brown, firm texture that will work with any tofu dish.

Chicken Tarragon with Couscous

We rarely eat chicken, but when we do, this dish is always a treat. Every now and then we share a craving for this seasoned and savory plate. The delicately flavored white-wine sauce makes a lively covering for the couscous. If you've never cooked couscous before, it can be remarkably simple to prepare, although the traditional Moroccan method is quite involved. We've happily settled for the packaged couscous, which is much quicker. If you can't find it in your local market, try a natural-foods or Greek market. Serve with Fresh Tomato Salad.

Serves 2.

1 Tbsp. canola oil
1 whole chicken breast, salted and
   peppered, then dipped in flour
2 cups mushrooms, sliced
1 tbsp. Wondra® flour
½ cup white wine
½ cup water
½ tsp. tarragon
Dash each of sugar, salt, pepper
2 cups dry couscous

In a large frying pan, heat the oil and sauté the chicken slowly until golden on all sides (about 15 minutes). Remove from the pan and keep warm. Add to the remaining oil the mushrooms and sauté until all liquid has evaporated. Add the white wine, water, flour, tarragon, sugar, salt, and pepper. Return the chicken breast to the pan and let simmer while covered for 20 minutes on low heat, or until chicken is done. Add a little water if necessary.

While the chicken simmers, prepare the couscous according to package directions.

Serve chicken over couscous, covered with mushroom sauce.

Chicken Fricassee
à la Berlin

German food is traditionally festive and comes in generous servings. Here the capers and asparagus add sharp flavor to this robust entree. Vegetables make this dish versatile, and it can easily become a vegetarian dish, substituting tofu for chicken and proceeding with the recipe in the same manner.

Serves 4.

2 whole chicken breasts, cut into chunks
   (1 lb. tofu for vegetarian version, drained
   and sliced into chunks)
1½ Tbsp. canola oil
1 onion, finely chopped
2 cups mushrooms, sliced
1 cup water
2 lb. asparagus tips or 1 15-oz. can green
   asparagus tips (save liquid)
3 Tbsp. Wondra® flour (it will not lump)
2 Tbsp. capers
Juice of ½ lemon
1 Tbsp. sugar
1 Tbsp. salt
1 tsp. pepper
1 Tbsp. fresh parsley, chopped

Heat oil in a medium-sized pot. Fry the onion until translucent. Add the mushrooms and fry until they turn light brown. Add the chicken and stir constantly while frying the chicken until it appears white on all sides, about 10 minutes.

Sprinkle flour over chicken and stir well. Then add the water, the asparagus and its juice, capers, lemon juice, sugar, salt, and pepper. Cook on low heat for 35 to 40 minutes, stirring occasionally. Just before serving sprinkle with parsley.

Serve hot over basmati rice or puff pastries.

Hunter Chicken Goulash

This dish is easily turned vegetarian by replacing the chicken with tofu. Either way, it is a hearty meal for a cold evening. Serve with Potato and Cucumber Salat. This is a typical Swabian Sunday meal.

Serves 2.

1½ Tbsp. canola oil
1 medium onion, finely chopped
½ lb. mushrooms, sliced
1 whole chicken breast without skin, cut
   into 1-inch cubes
1 Tbsp. tomato paste
1 package Knorr® Hunter Sauce Mix or
   Brown Gravy Mix
2 cups water (1 cup to be used for sauce
   mix)
½ cup beer (optional)
Salt, pepper, and sugar to taste

Salt and pepper the chicken.

Heat oil on high heat and sauté onion until golden brown. Add mushrooms and stir frequently until they are brown and all liquid has evaporated. When the mushrooms begin to smoke, add chicken pieces and stir for 2 minutes. Add tomato paste and stir. Remove from heat.

Combine sauce mix with 1 cup water, stir well, and add to the chicken. Follow with other cup of water, the beer (optional) and simmer for 35 minutes. Add salt, pepper, and sugar to taste. Consistency should be creamy.

Serve hot over wide noodles.

Pollo All'Arrabbiata

Baked in a cooking bag, surrounded by fresh and spicy tomato sauce, this chicken is delicious. It's easy to make, and you can prepare extra sauce for Penne All'Arrabbiata later in the week.

Serves 2–4.

2 chicken breasts without skin
2 Tbsp. flour
Sauce All'Arrabbiata
1 Reynolds® cooking bag, 14 × 20 inches

Prepare All'Arrabbiata sauce according to recipe, but simmer only 10 minutes.

Drop flour into cooking bag, followed by All'Arrabbiata sauce. Add the chicken breasts. Turn the bag carefully to coat chicken and seal with a nylon tie. Slice four small slits in the top of the bag and place in a casserole dish. Bake at 350° for 40 minutes, or until tender.

Serve chicken and sauce over a plate of pasta.

Kasha Varnishkes

A simple variation on an old classic, easy to prepare and always satisfying. Kasha is the Russian word for buckwheat, loaded with protein and vitamins. Grandma used to prepare this meal on special holidays and occasions, but we think it's too tasty and too easy to make to save for only special treats.

Serves 2 (or more if served as a side dish).

2 cups bow-tie noodles
1 cup whole roasted kasha kernels
2 cups water
½ tsp. salt
Dash pepper
1 onion, chopped
1 tsp. butter

Combine water, salt, and pepper in a small saucepan and bring to a boil. Add the kasha and reduce the heat to simmer for about 10 minutes.

While the kasha cooks, melt the butter in a small frying pan and add the onion, stirring until brown. Add to the kasha.

Prepare 2 cups of bow-tie noodles according to directions on package.

Mix the kasha with the noodles and serve hot.

Potato Pancakes Eleonore

*Grandma was wise enough
to know we couldn't wait
until Chanukah time for
these traditional treats!
These "latkes" were as big a
part of my childhood as
stickball and Coney Island.
We still make them, following Granny's recipe, which
her grandmother made for
her when she was a child.
In our family we've made a
ritual of preparing the
quintessential latke: on top
of the pancake place a
spoonful of sour cream (we
use nonfat), or an equally
generous scoop of fresh (still
warm) applesauce. Our
daughter stands by the combination of sour cream AND
applesauce.*

Serves 2.

**5 medium potatoes, peeled and finely
    grated**
2 eggs
½ onion, finely grated
1 tsp. salt
2 Tbsp. canola oil

Grate the potatoes in a large, very fine
strainer and rinse with cold water. Drain off
all liquid and add the onion. This should
be a pastelike mass. Put the mixture in a
medium-sized bowl and add the eggs and
salt.

Heat the oil in a frying pan. Drop into pan a
heaping spoonful of the potato mixture, flat-
tened like a pancake, and fry until crunchy
golden brown. Place the cooked pancakes on
a short stack of folded paper towels to remove the excess oil.

Serve the pancakes hot with fresh applesauce and/or light sour cream.

Quick applesauce:
4 tart apples (Granny Smith, if available)
1 Tbsp. honey

Peel the apples and remove their cores.
Cook the apples whole in 2 cups boiling
water for 15 minutes or until very soft. Add
the honey and mash well.

Potato Pirogen

Here's a low-fat version of
another recipe from
Grandma's kitchen. It's simple and inexpensive to prepare and simply a delight to
eat. Although these small
pastries are traditionally
served as an appetizer, we
think they are hearty
enough to be a main dish,
especially when served with
a light salad, like the Fresh
Tomato Salad.

Serves 4.

Step 1—dough:
2 eggs
½ cup water
3 cups flour, sifted
½ tsp. salt

Beat eggs and water, sift flour and salt together, and combine gradually. Ingredients
should make a firm dough. Cover and let
stand for 20 minutes.

Step 2—filling:
**4 medium potatoes, peeled, cubed and
    boiled until very soft**
½ cup parsley, finely chopped
1 large onion, chopped
1 teaspoon canola oil
1 Tbsp. Maggi
1 tsp. salt
Pinch pepper

Brown the onions in oil over high heat.
Mash the potatoes until creamy and add
parsley, onion, Maggi, salt, and pepper to
taste.

Step 3:
Divide dough into two portions. Roll out
with a rolling pin until ¼-inch thick. Cut
into rounds about 4 to 5 inches in diameter
using the rim of a glass or a round cookie
cutter. Fill each round with 1 tsp. potato
mixture. Seal edges with egg white to hold
them together.

Step 4:
Drop pierogies in boiling salted water and
cook for 10 minutes or until they rise to the
top of the pot. Serve hot with nonfat sour
cream and a tiny bit of butter.

Matzoh Brie

Tried and true, this dish is a simple pleasure that brings smiles to their faces every time it's served . . . at breakfast or dinner. This Jewish recipe is customarily served during Passover, but like so many of my grandmother's traditional recipes, it is too tasty to reserve only for holidays. Matzoh Brie inspires a warm and traditional mood no matter what time of the year it is served. Delicious with Green Bean Salat.

Serves 2.

4 cups warm water
8 slices of plain matzoh
3 egg whites and 1 yolk
6 oz. skim milk
½ tsp. salt
¼ tsp. pepper
1 Tbsp. canola oil

Break up the matzoh in a large mixing bowl and let it soak in warm water for 5 minutes.

Whisk together egg whites and milk.

Drain the water from the matzoh and add the milk-and-egg mixture. Let stand for 5 minutes.

Heat oil in a large frying pan. Add the matzoh mixture. Sprinkle with salt and pepper. Cook over medium flame, turning and stirring frequently, until crunchy and lightly browned.

Spinach and Mashed Potatoes

This truly homemade German dish is a favorite in our house. It's quick to make and loaded with valuable nutrients and protein.

Serves 2.

Potatoes:
2 medium potatoes, peeled
1 tsp. salt
1 tsp. pepper
½ cup skim milk
1 tsp. butter

Cut the peeled potatoes into small pieces and boil until very soft. Drain, and add butter, milk, salt and pepper. Mash thoroughly and keep warm.

Spinach:
3 bunches fresh spinach, or 1 package
  frozen creamed spinach
1 cup water
½ tsp. salt
4 eggs

While potatoes cook, prepare the spinach.

Boil the eggs until hard. Remove and discard the yolks and chop the egg whites. Keep the chopped egg whites warm.

If you are using fresh spinach, clean it well, remove the stems, and boil until soft. Drain the water and empty the spinach into a blender and chop well. If you are using frozen spinach, prepare according to directions on package.

Mix the chopped spinach with the mashed potatoes, add the chopped eggs, and serve warm.

Readings and References

The Triumphant Patient by Greg Anderson, Nelson. 1992.
(For cancer patients and those that love them)

Beyond the Relaxation Response by Herbert Benson. Times Books. 1984.
(This Harvard physician is the academic spirit of the entire wellness movement)

Inner Joy by Harold Blookfield and Richard Kory. Wynden. 1983.
(A healing psychiatrist shows how)

Wholeness and Implicate Order by David Bohm. Routledge and Kegan, Paul, 1980.
(A Nobel Prize winning physicist explains purpose and meaning)

Fire in the Soul by Joan Borysenko. Warner Books, 1993.
(Powerful spiritual answers to modern problems)

Healing the Shame that Binds You by John Bradshaw. Health Communications, 1988.
(For alcoholics and those who love them)

A Dancing Star by Eileen Campbell. Aquarian Press, 1991.
(A marvelous collection of inspirational quotations)

Ageless Body, Timeless Mind by Deepak Chopra. Harmony, 1993.
(An eminent physician shares breathtaking truths)

Anatomy of an Illness by Norman Cousins. Norton, 1979. Bantam, 1981.
(The beginning of Mind Body Medicine)

The Mind of God by Paul Davies. Touchstone, 1992.
(An astronomer labels humanity as "animated stardust")

Fit for Life by Harvey and Marilyn Diamond. Warner Books, 1985.
(Deservedly the best selling nutrition book, ever)

Healing Words by Larry Dossey. HarperCollins, 1993.
(An eminent physician explores the scientific basis of healing prayer)

Real Magic by Wayne Dyer. HarperCollins, 1992.
(True healing alchemy)

The World as I See It by Albert Einstein. Citadel, 1978.
(The genius discusses the meaning and nobility of life)

Man's Search for Meaning by Viktor E. Frankl. Washington Square Press, 1959
(A psychiatrist survives a concentration camp with unwavering faith)

Love's Labor by Stanley E. Greben. Schocken Books, 1984.
    (A psychiatrist to love)

The Dancing Healers by Carl A. Hammerschlag. HarperCollins, 1988.
    (A physician's journey of healing with American Indians)

Healing from Within by Dennis T. Jaffe. Bantam Books, 1980.
    (Readable, touching and informative)

Love Is Letting Go of Fear by Gerald G. Jampolsky. Celestial Arts, 1979.
    (A psychiatrist who teaches only love)

Avalanche by W. Brugh Joy. Ballantine Books, 1990.
    (Experience an inner mental and spiritual avalanche)

Who Gets Sick by Blair Justice. Tarcher, 1988.
    (Chronicles the sociology and mass psychology of illness)

Giant Steps by Barry N. Kaufman. Fawcett, 1979.
    (Reveals that happiness is a choice—and explains how to choose it)

Peace of Mind by Joshua Loth Liebman. Simon and Schuster, 1946.
    (A Rabbi for now!)

Toward a Psychology of Being by Abraham H. Maslow. Van Nostrand Reinhold, 1968.
    (Liberation from Freud and the beginning of understanding)

Care of the Soul by Thomas Moore. HarperCollins, 1993.
    (A brilliant, extraordinary work whose title says it all)

Healing and the Mind by Bill Moyers. Doubleday, 1993
    (A comprehensive survey of the connections between the mind and the body)

Eat More, Weigh Less by Dean Ornish. HarperCollins, 1993.
    (A physician successfully challenges the establishment and makes history!)

Further Along the Road Less Travelled by M. Scott Peck. Simon and Schuster, 1993.
    (An extremely worthwhile update of a modern classic)

Mind As Healer, Mind As Slayer by Kenneth R. Pellitier. Delacorte Press, 1977.
    (A brilliant explanation of how we become sick)

Sai Baba, The Holy Man and The Psychiatrist by Samuel H. Sandweiss. Birthday Press, 1975.
(A psychiatrist explores his spiritual love)

Power Thoughts by Robert Schuller. HarperCollins, 1993.
(Powerful wisdom for powerful thinkers)

Love, Medicine and Miracles by Bernie S. Siegel. HarperCollins, 1986.
(A psychician offers touching wisdom for health and well being)

Getting Well Again by O. Carl Simonton, Stephanie Matthews-Simonton, and James Creighton. J.P. Tarcher, 1978. Bantam, 1980.
(The classic work of a pioneering physician offering hope for cancer patients)

The Wisdom of the Ego by George E. Vaillant. Harvard, 1993.
(For academics, this is the Harvard way)

A Return to Love by Marianne Williamson. HarperCollins, 1992.
(A minister brings love and forgiveness closer to home)

Spiritual Diary by Parmahansa Yogananda. Self Realization Fellowship, 1977.
(A classic for our time)

Cookbooks:

A Taste of Heaven and Earth by Bettina Vitell. Harper Perennial, 1993.

American Vegetarian Cookbook by Marilyn Diamond. Warner Books, 1990.

Gourmet Vegetarian Feasts by Martha Rose Shulman. Thorsons, 1984.

Simply Vegetarian by the Cooks of Ananda. Crystal Clarity, 1989.

The Enchanted Broccoli Forest by Mollie Katzen. Ten Speed Press, 1982.

The Gradual Vegetarian by Lisa Tracy. Evans Publishers, 1985.

The Greens Cookbook by Deborah Madison and Edward E. Brown. Bantam Books, 1987.

The Inspired Vegetarian by Louise Pickford. Stewart Tabori and Chang, 1992.

The Moosewood Cookbook by Mollie Katzen. Ten Speed Press, 1977.

The Top One Hundred Pasta Sauces by Diane Seed. Ten Speed Press, 1987.

Special Request
and Additional Resources

CORRESPONDENCE

Dr. Taub greatly appreciates receiving letters from readers willing to share their experiences and describe the effects of the Wellness Rx. Your information is important to ongoing clinical research. Please address your letters to The Wellness Medicine Institute, Box #82, Mt. Carmel, IL 62863.

MEDITATION TAPES

Dr. Taub has recorded a special audiotape to induce a state of deep relaxation and meditation in adults and children (ages 4–14). He has also created an entire album, "The Seven-Day Stress Relief System," containing eight different meditation audiotapes. If you wish to purchase any of these tapes or the album, please write to The Wellness Medicine Institute, Box #82, Mt. Carmel, IL 62863. Each individual tape is $12 and the album is $60. These prices *include* postage and handling. Please make checks payable to The Wellness Medicine Institute.

#1 Relaxation and Healing Meditation Tape
#2 Relaxation and Healing Meditation for children (ages 4–14)
#3 The Seven-Day Stress Relief System Album (includes tape #1)

QUIT SMOKING PROGRAM

Doctor Taub is a spokesperson and medical consultant for *The National Wellness Stop Smoking Campaign*. This powerful program supported by the American Medical Association is the largest smoking cessation initiative in history. Dr. Taub highly recommends the program's comprehensive "How to Quit" smoker's kit, containing an instructional video, relaxation audiotapes, and other special aids for smoking cessation. The smoker's kit is available by request from: The Wellness Medicine Institute, Box #82, Mt. Carmel, IL 62863.

Index